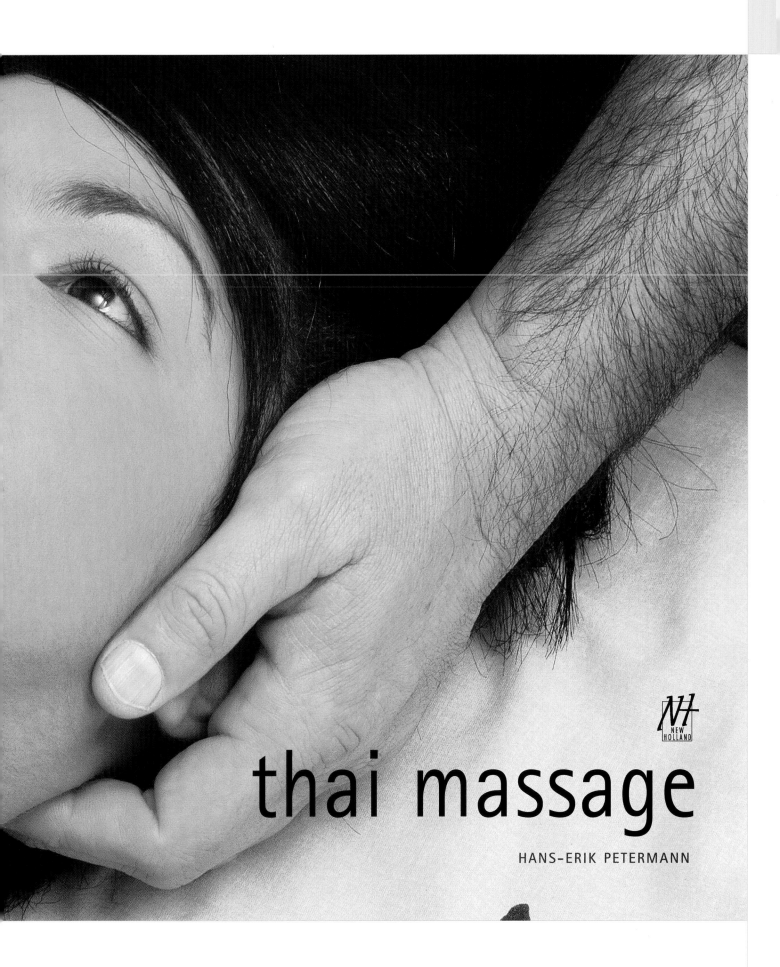

NH
NEW
HOLLAND

thai massage

HANS-ERIK PETERMANN

First published in 2006 by New Holland Publishers Ltd

London • Cape Town • Sydney • Auckland

www.newhollandpublishers.com

86 Edgware Road, London W2 2EA, United Kingdom • 80 McKenzie Street, Cape Town 8001, South Africa • 14 Aquatic Drive, Frenchs Forest, NSW 2086, Australia • 218 Lake Road, Northcote, Auckland, New Zealand

ISBN 1 84537 035 X (hardback)

ISBN 1 84537 036 8 (paperback)

Publisher and editor: Mariëlle Renssen

Publishing Managers: Claudia Dos Santos, Simon Pooley

Commissioning editor: Alfred LeMaitre

Designer: Steven Felmore

Picture research: Karla Kik, Tamlyn McGeean

Illustrations: Steven Felmore

Production: Myrna Collins

Consultant: Simon Gall, School Principal,
   London School of Thai Massage, UK

Reproduction by Resolution Colour (Pty) Ltd, Cape Town

Printed and bound in Malaysia by Times Offset (M) Sdn. Bhd

10 9 8 7 6 5 4 3 2 1

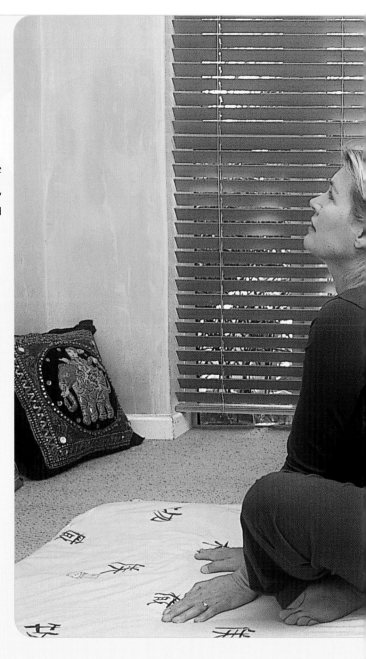

DISCLAIMER

Although the author and publishers have made every effort to ensure that the information contained in this book was accurate at the time of going to press, they accept no responsibility for any loss, injury, or inconvenience sustained by any person using this book or following the advice given in it.

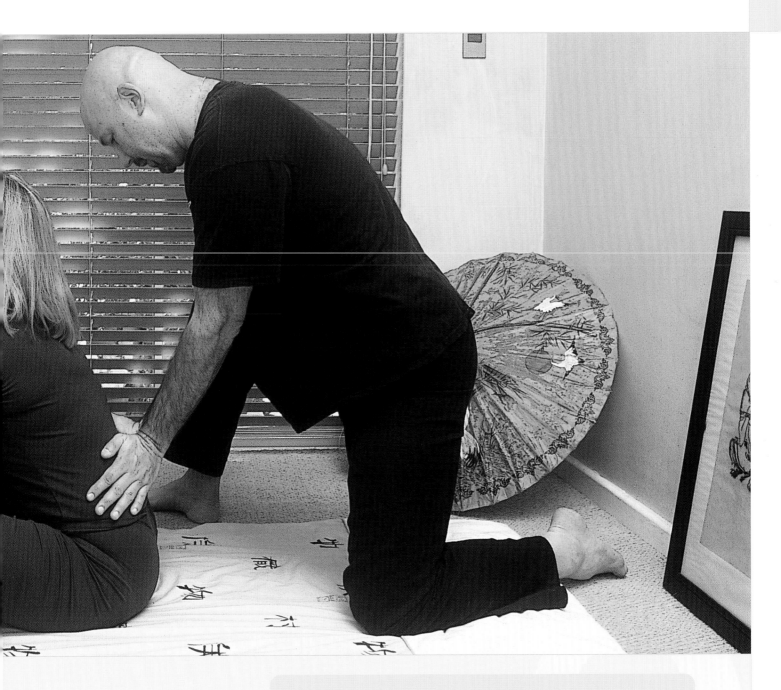

DEDICATION

To my parents, for supporting me in realizing my dreams.
And to Janet — I wish she were here to read this book.

AUTHOR'S ACKNOWLEDGEMENTS

My grateful thanks to Chongkol Setthakorn, master teacher of Thai massage,
and to all of the massage therapists in Thailand who so generously shared
their knowledge with me.

part one

History and development, East vs. West, underlying
principles of Thai massage. Role of the therapist.
Exercises and meditations.

part two

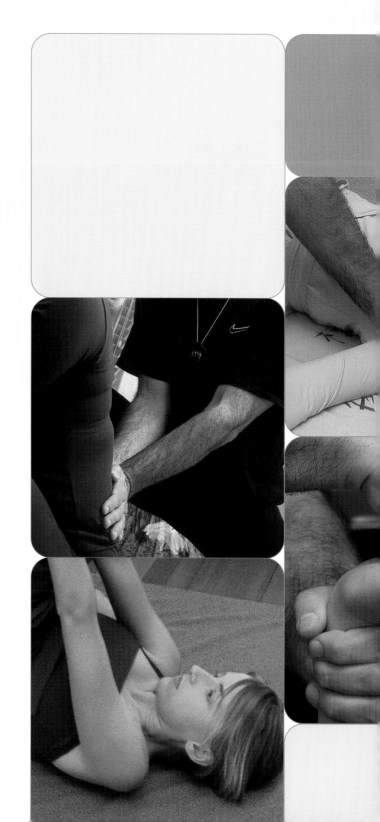

Contents

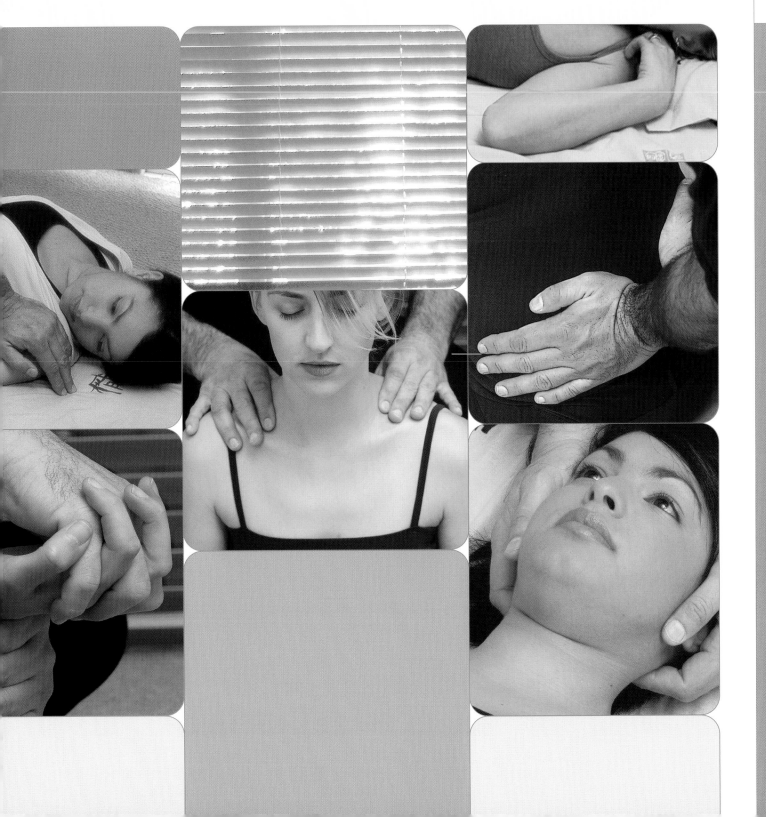

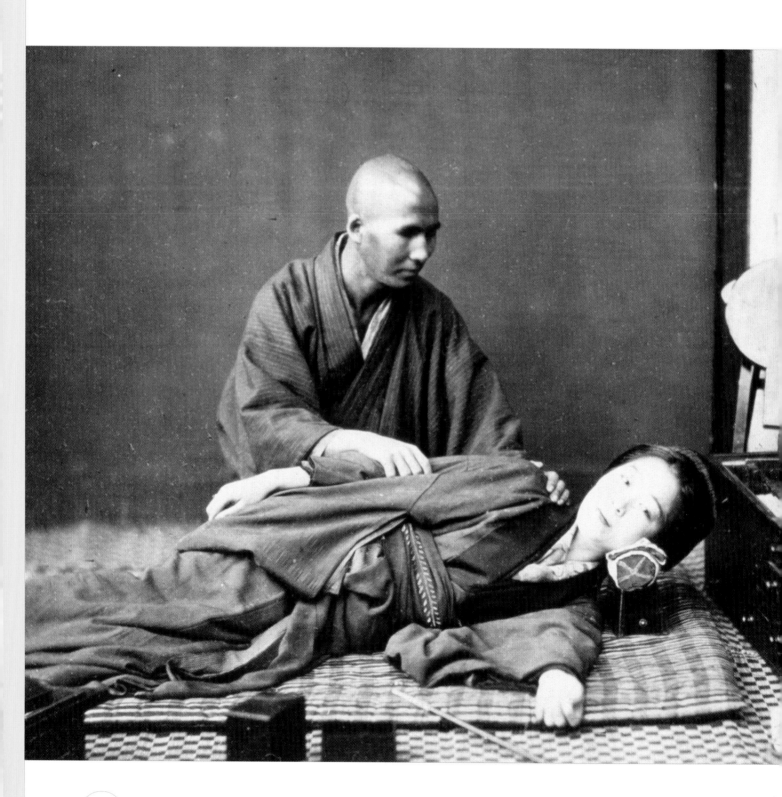

Part One
What is Thai massage?

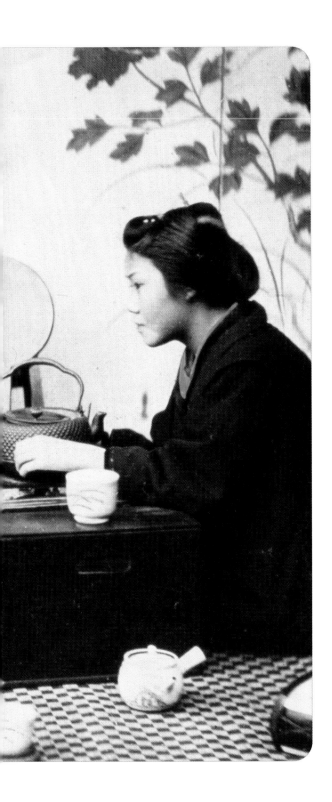

MASSAGE, IN ONE FORM OR ANOTHER, HAS BEEN IN EXISTENCE for thousands of years. Archaeological finds going back to ancient India, Egypt and Greece, such as painted reliefs and clay jars, clearly show distinct bodywork techniques being used in ancient times. Physicians in ancient Greece wrote books on the subject. Julius Caesar's biographer, Caius Seutonius Tranquillus, in *Lives of the Twelve Caesars*, mentions the daily massages the Roman leader received. The touching and rubbing of an aching body in all probability goes back to the first cave-dwelling mother applying loving physical touch to her child. The need for touch, for bodily contact and warmth is basic to all human beings, as well as to many animal species.

Healers of the past from any social group tended to be those who had a special aptitude and sensitivity for the task. They in turn passed on the skills of a lifetime to the next generation. Over time it would become clear that certain patterns of disease tended to repeat themselves and could be treated by specific massage techniques or routines. From generation to generation this knowledge was refined, codified and passed on.

This, then, is the origin of the distinctive types of bodywork used today. Each system of massage tended to be a reflection of the environment and culture out of which it arose.

In the West, in European culture as it has developed over the last few centuries, the dominant world-view has been the scientific, rational one, and it has shaped every aspect of this

Left This albumen print (c.1890) by Felice Beato (1825–c.1908) of a Japanese shiatsu session is evidence of the popularity of massage therapies in the East in earlier times.

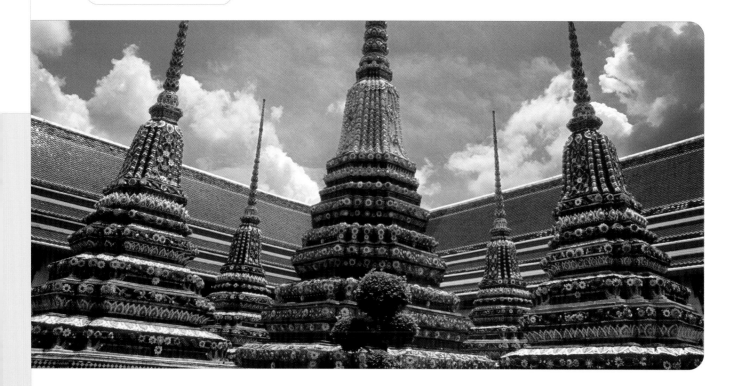

culture. The healer, whether a doctor, bonesetter or massage therapist, is perceived to be carrying out his work on an uninformed, passive client. In Asian healing modalities, there tends to be more of a belief in the necessity for the therapist to work together with the client, where there is a corresponding sense of awareness. Treatment is centred less on elements of the physical structure and more on harmonizing the flow of the vital energy seen as the basis for all life. This vital energy — or 'life force' — goes by different names in different Asian cultures, but, conceptually, it is fairly identical from one culture to the next. In India it is referred to as 'prana', in China it is called 'chi' and in Japan 'ki'.

While all forms of massage by definition use physical techniques to achieve their aim, the great difference between the European and Asian massage traditions mirrors the differences in culture and world-view. Nearly every Asian country has its own tradition of bodywork, and the better known of these traditions are Japanese shiatsu, Chinese acupressure and Indian Ayurvedic massage.

In the last few decades, the beauty of Thailand's landscape and culture and the hospitality of the Thai people have led to millions of tourists visiting that country. As a result, many of them have experienced the wellbeing gained from a gentle

Thai massage — and many of these people have subsequently studied this massage system and brought it back with them to their own countries. In this way, Thai massage has become available, and very popular, all over the world.

Massage systems usually tend to be oriented toward either working on the structure of the body or on its energy systems. In recent times, with the spread of knowledge from all cultures, massage systems have come into being that attempt to integrate the structural work with the energy work. Massage, or bodywork, can be defined as a treatment in which the therapist uses various parts of his or her body, usually predominantly the hands, to exert pressure, cause friction or move the limbs of the client's body. This is done with the aim of creating a feeling of wellbeing; or integrating or improving the client's physical structure or energy system (or both); or even changing a state of disease to one of health. Whatever the theoretical orientation of each massage system may be, they all are aimed at improving the health and wellbeing of the client. A good Thai

Above **The Thai massage tradition is infused with Buddhist influences. Here, Wat Phra Keo, part of Bangkok's Temple of the Emerald Buddha, is typical of the beautiful, intricately adorned Buddhist structures.**

massage, completely based as it is on an energy-oriented model, will still improve blood circulation, promote postural integration and a greater range of motion around the major joints. Conversely, a good Swedish massage, in improving the circulation of blood and lymph fluids, and creating more relaxed, efficient breathing, will have a positive impact on the subtle energy flows of the client. The Western vs. Eastern, 'structure vs. energy' discussion is important in understanding how the different methods work, but in the case of very experienced and sensitive massage therapists, positive results will be experienced in every dimension of the client's bodily health.

The **skeletal system** is composed of bones and cartilage. In so far as there is skeletal misalignment — in the spine, for instance — this can be rectified, whether by some of the Eastern-oriented spinal rotational stretches of Thai massage or by the more vigorous adjustments of Western chiropractic.

The **muscular system**, in which the muscles facilitate physical movement, makes up about 40 per cent of body weight. Release of tension brought about by Swedish massage promotes more efficient movement as much as the release brought about by a shiatsu or Thai massage stretch.

The **circulatory system** benefits from all forms of massage as it improves the circulation of blood and lymph through the body, removing toxic wastes and supplying nutrients and oxygen to the cells.

The **nervous system**, which controls the functioning of the entire body, benefits from massage in that it becomes more balanced. It is either stimulated or sedated by the massage techniqe, whichever is necessary at the time.

The **respiratory system** — our breathing mechanism — is also harmonized by a good massage as breathing slows down and deepens, bringing more oxygen into the lungs. And both the **digestive** and **urinary systems** benefit in that the functions of the organs, such as the liver and kidney, are positively affected, and the elimination of waste materials and toxins becomes more efficient.

So, in summary, although the above results are common to most effective massages, it is the conceptual understanding of how and why the body benefits from massage that marks the greatest difference between the West's more structure-oriented approach and Asia's more energy-based systems.

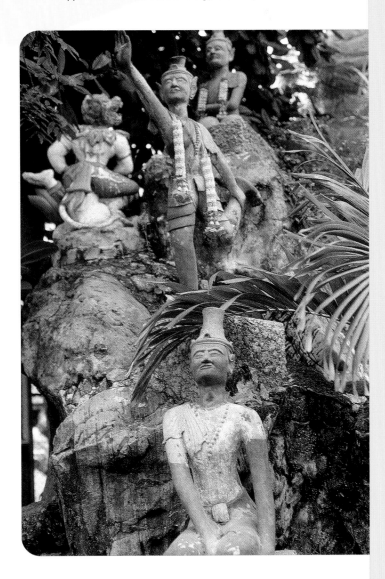

Right Within the grounds of the royal temple, Wat Po, in Bangkok are a number of statues representing various aspects of the traditional Thai massage that is taught in the temple school based here.

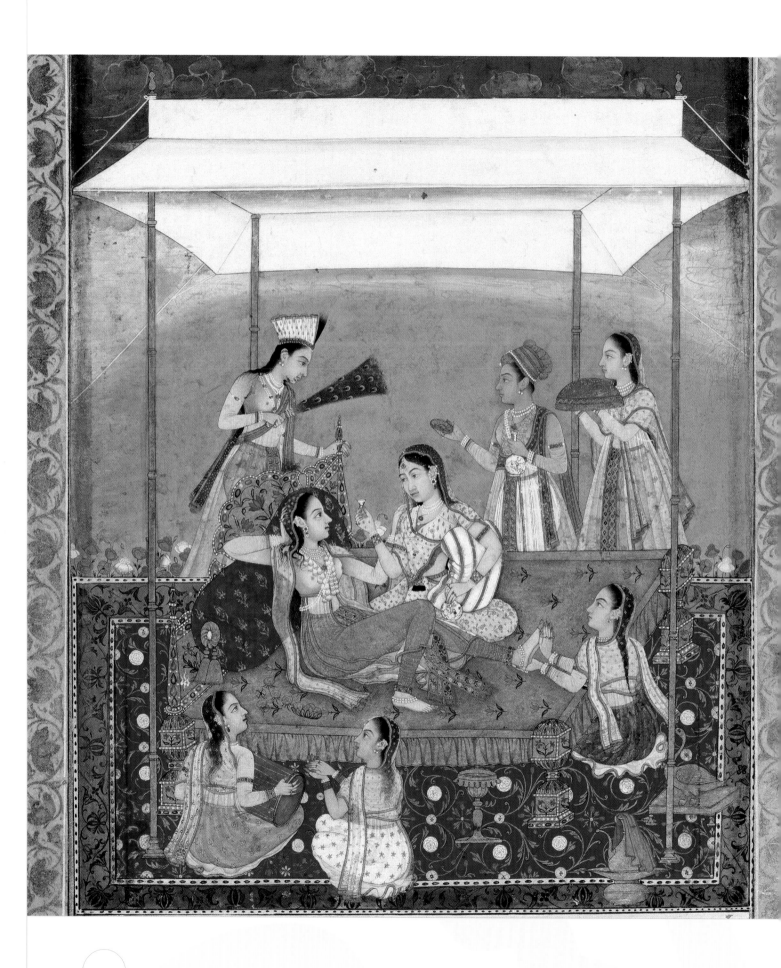

EASTERN ATTITUDES VS. WESTERN

IN DRAWING TOGETHER THOUSANDS OF YEARS OF HISTORY and development in Europe and Asia in a brief comparative overview, it's necessary to generalize. Broad cultural beliefs form the basis for the understanding of health, disease and medical care. In the West, there has been great faith in the 'infallibility' of science — we believe what our physical senses tell us. Stronger microscopes or improved chemical analyses give us better information and therefore greater understanding. A state of disease manifests itself through symptoms; by grouping these symptoms together, a doctor is able to reach a reasonably accurate assumption as to what type of disease or medical problem he or she is confronted with. Having established what the problem is, there are specific definitive solutions: for example, realign the vertebrae, remove the diseased organ or take tablets to re-establish chemical balance in the body. It's a very linear, logical and well-defined process. It also implies a healer who knows what the problem is and can solve it, and a patient or client who is medically ignorant and therefore passive.

There is a clear separation between a medical doctor — 'all-knowing' and near 'infallible' — and other types of healers who are often considered, at best, as support staff in the fight against disease. Indeed, in some cases, medicine may well be the optimal approach! By the time an artery is blocked and a heart attack imminent, it might be a little late to think in terms of energy balancing, lifestyle changes and stress-relieving practices such as yoga or tai chi. At this point, surgical intervention and a triple bypass may be the only means of preventing the client's death.

The Eastern medical model sees things somewhat differently. Traditionally, in China, it sometimes happened that a doctor would receive regular payment to keep a client healthy. If the client fell ill, the regular payment would stop. Prevention thus meant everything; having to cope with an advanced state of disease signified failure as a practitioner. The means by which a healer kept track of the client's health was by sensitively monitoring the flow of vital energy through the body. This vital energy, which cannot be measured by the instruments of Western science, is believed to flow through certain pathways in the human body called 'meridians' in acupuncture, *nadi* in Ayurvedic medicine and *sen* in Thai massage. To the accusation that what cannot be seen or measured does not exist, the ever-pragmatic Chinese medical doctors would demonstrate how, for instance, acupuncture needles alone could be used for the purposes of anaesthesia in a surgical operation. The idea was that, if it worked — and did so repeatedly — they would continue using this method. Their conceptual rationale was simply based on a philosophy or world-view that might not be clear to the Western mind. In the Asian world-view, everything in the universe is part of the ebb and flow of universal energy. When this flow is balanced, and harmonious, all is well; when there is stagnation or imbalance, problems of wellbeing arise.

The energy flow within the human body can be analogous to the road system of any city. There are bigger roads as a result

Left An 18th-century watercolour painting by the Mughal School depicts a lady in a pretty garden setting being treated to a foot massage, to the accompaniment of music. The artwork hangs in the Victoria and Albert Museum, London.

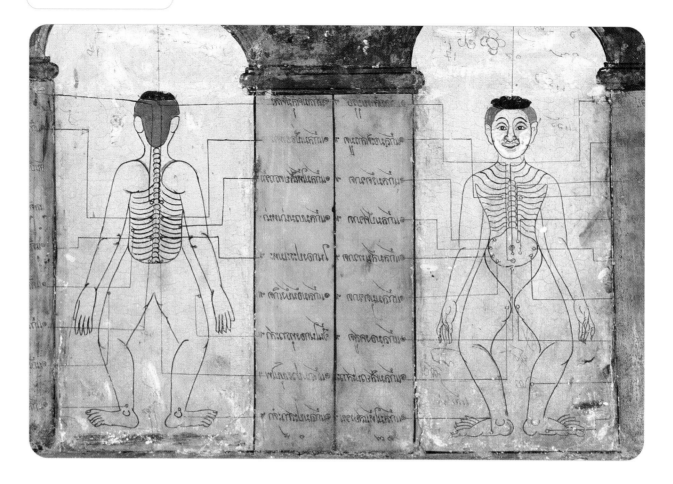

of what they are connecting, and smaller country roads. There are intersections through which a lot of traffic flows. Should there be an accident or a blockage at a major intersection, the traffic backs up and, given sufficient time, slows down to a crawl; the result is that your blood pressure rises.

Bearing this analogy in mind, in an energy-based Asian medical system, the doctor or healer will monitor the energy flow. The more sensitive the healer, the earlier he will pick up imbalances, blockages or stagnation. Should there be deviation from the normal balanced flow, the healer will use the tools at his disposal to re-establish a harmonious, balanced flow. These tools might include, but would not necessarily be limited to, acupuncture, moxibustion (see below), herbal remedies, changing the client's nutritional patterns, and bodywork or massage. (Moxibustion is a Chinese method of treatment in which burning plant material is held close to the skin, the heat acting as a cauterizing agent or skin counterirritant.)

Seen from this broader perspective, the differences become clear. In the West, you are perfectly healthy until you have a group of identifiable, coherent symptoms, at which point you are already sick and need a doctor to mend the malfunction. In the Eastern view, there is less of a sharp delineation between health and disease. Your energy flow is rarely either totally balanced or seriously out of kilter, rather somewhere in-between, so generally a good massage is all you may need to make you feel a little healthier. It's a part of your natural health maintenance, thus a good massage therapist is seen as no less valuable a member of the community of healers than the Ayurvedic surgeon or the Chinese acupuncturist.

Above These 19th-century wall paintings executed by the Thai School are representations of Eastern-based energy lines and massage points on the human body. The paintings appear on the walls of the temple, Wat Po, in Bangkok, Thailand.

HOW DIFFERENT IS THAI MASSAGE?

Origins and influences

All of the better known Asian bodywork, or massage, systems (Chinese acupressure, Ayurvedic massage and Japanese shiatsu) are based on energy flow and, to some extent, share similarities with Thai massage. It may be useful to look at this in a comparative historical context.

We can make our point by, for instance, seeing India as having played a key role in early Asian civilization. It is from India that the Buddhist missionary monks travelled to China, Japan and Southeast Asia, bringing with them not only their religion but also their medical knowledge and even martial arts techniques. Wherever they settled and propagated their faith, they also passed on their medical and martial knowledge. Over the centuries, this knowledge would fuse with the local traditions and culture, creating something different and new. Yet at its core it clearly shared the same roots.

In China, for instance, Buddhism interacted with Taoist mysticism to form Chan Buddhism, which became better known in the West by its Japanese name, Zen Buddhism. The Indian martial arts were transformed into Shaolin Kung Fu. Thousands of years later it has become close to impossible to disentangle exactly what part of the vast field of Chinese medical knowledge has Indian origins and what existed prior to the fusion with Indian knowledge.

Although Thai massage has similarities with other major Asian massage systems, it is in many ways unique. Yes, it is energy-based as are the other Asian systems. It utilizes 10 main energy lines known as *sen*. The *sen* are drawn from the Indian Ayurvedic medical tradition, which refers to 72,000 energy lines (or *nadis*) in the human body. (Although far beyond the scope of this book, it is possible to speculate that these pretty much cover every possible energy line in the

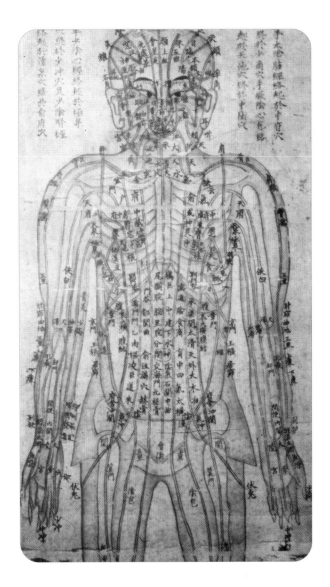

human body, including the meridians.) All 10 *sen* from Thai massage are connected to the energy centre of the body – the abdomen area – and connect up to the sensory organs and the zones of the body concerned with elimination. These lines are not identical to the acupuncture/acupressure meridians used in Chinese massage or in Japanese shiatsu, which are all related to specific organs.

A strong Indian influence in Thai massage is also clearly indicated in its large component of yoga-type stretches. Shiatsu uses some stretching techniques, acupressure less so.

Right **An ancient chart shows the Chinese version of acupuncture and energy lines of the body.**

STRUCTURAL VS. INTUITIVE APPROACH

There is an apparent lack of deep theoretical structure to Thai massage. In the major massage schools in Thailand today, a great number of techniques are taught but there is little in the way of specific diagnosis of problems and definite cures to such problems — although there *are* specific treatments for particular problems. Much is left to the intuition of the practitioner and the strong overall balancing effect a treatment has on the energy system as a whole.

In shiatsu, by contrast, there are four specific methods of diagnosis: *bo shin* (visual assessment), *bun shin* (assessment of the client's speech and bodily odour), *mon shin* (questioning the client directly) and *setsu shin* (assessing via manual touch). Energy can be excessive (*jitsu*) or deficient (*kyo*). In combination with the meridians and the theory of the five elements, this is a far more detailed system of diagnosis and treatment.

Some use this conceptual sophistication to make a case for shiatsu as a true medical massage system while Thai massage is viewed at best as a more generalized 'pick-me-up' treatment. Certainly, the more systematized a treatment is, the easier it may be to teach, especially to beginners. Many Thai practitioners, on the other hand, feel this is not true. Since the work with the energy system is so intuitive, they believe the creation of too many set, pre-existing categories may be

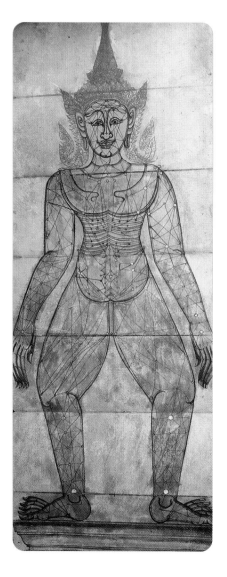

limiting rather than useful, especially to the beginner or intermediate level practitioner, as it prevents him or her from approaching the client with an attitude of open, sensitive awareness. In other words, instead of quiet, focused listening, one is trying to find the right category into which to place the client. It's possible, too, that the highly organized nature of shiatsu reflects the psyche of the Japanese culture within which it operates; in this respect, Thai culture is more open, more relaxed and possibly more intuitive.

Another reason for the apparent lack of recorded theoretical knowledge is that many of the classical texts on the subject were destroyed during the Burmese invasion in 1769.

In the end, though, such comparisons might only be of academic interest. Faced with a severely imbalanced energy flow in a client, an experienced master of either of these two forms of massage is able to re-establish harmony and balance. Each will simply go about it in a slightly different way. Western students will, depending on their personality, prefer the structure of the one or the other.

Above **Every Eastern culture has its own interpretation of the energy centres and pressure points used in a diversity of massage techniques; this artwork is of Thai origin.**

TAKING UP THAI MASSAGE

Known in Thailand as *nuad bo rarn*, or *nuad phan bo rarn*, Thai massage traces its origins back to India, to a physician called Shivago Komarpaj. This Ayurvedic doctor is reputed to have treated even Buddha himself, and he is regarded as the 'father' of all Thai medical knowledge, not just its massage system.

It is unfortunate that most of the written records of the Thai medical tradition existing at the time were destroyed some 2000 years later during a Burmese invasion in 1769. Many decades later, ruling monarch King Rama III (1824–51) commissioned the carving of the material that had been saved onto the walls of Wat Po temple in Bangkok.

Historically there is a strong connection between Buddhist beliefs and Thai massage — to the degree that many teachers maintain the core of a good Thai massage to be *metta*, the Buddhist practice of loving kindness. This doesn't mean that any aspiring Thai massage therapist has to adopt a Buddhist belief system. It simply means that Thai, and any other kind of massage, is best given in a spirit of loving kindness. Such a spirit lies at the core of most of the major world religions.

While there are larger massage schools in Thailand, a lot of the teaching has traditionally been passed down from teachers to small numbers of students. As a result of this, quite a large number of techniques and variations have been created over the centuries.

Today there are two styles of Thai massage in existence: the Southern and the Northern styles, with a number of differences between them.

Southern-style massages, especially as taught at Wat Po, tend to be shorter in duration; the Northern-style massages may be up to two or three hours long. The Southern style also tends not to use as many stretching techniques, making use rather of a vigorous 'twanging', or 'plucking', of the tendons and along some of the energy lines.

However, in recent years there has been an increasing tendency to amalgamate the two styles, as people have been learning the techniques of both.

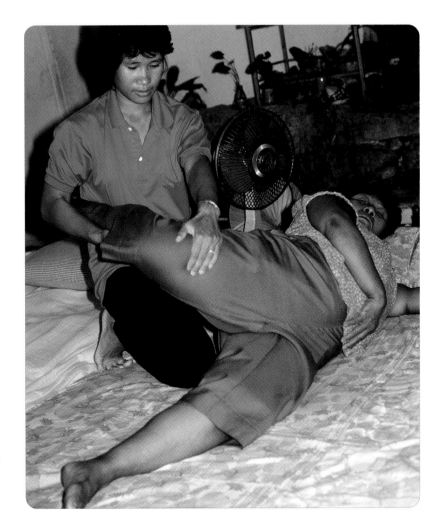

Right In Thailand, legwork is the focus of any massage session because of hours spent on foot and working in the fields.

Altogether there are probably several hundred techniques in Thai massage, if one includes all the variations in the count. While all these techniques should be learned and mastered over time if you wish to consider yourself a fully qualified Thai massage therapist, it is initially probably better to learn a limited and thus more manageable selection of techniques that are useful for a general treatment. If you want to pursue further studies, it is strongly recommended that you find yourself a teacher. Although some techniques can be learned from a book, possibly together with practice sessions on a friend, this is only the beginning of the learning process.

The selection of techniques for this book was done on the basis of creating a standardized one-hour session that would promote balanced energy flow in the whole body, and it includes most of the basic techniques. The average client who won't have come across Thai massage performed in a holiday setting usually can't afford more than an hour, timewise. Where most books attempt to show the full range of tech-niques, this is potentially too much for a beginner to absorb if studying on his or her own, and is not necessary for a one-

hour treatment. By using this shortened form of massage as a basic study, the aspiring therapist can then fully enjoy learning the great number of variations and advanced techniques at a later stage.

In modern Western culture, most accumulated stress tends to manifest itself in the neck and shoulders, in which case a massage routine would focus fairly extensively on this area, with the client seated upright in a cross-legged position. The traditional routine, however, begins with the client lying on his back, and as much as half of the massage may be taken up by work done on the legs. The reason for this is that Thailand was (and is) traditionally an agricultural society and most of the work was done manually, even in the cities. Also, only a small percentage of the population owns a motor vehicle. Thus, the legs are the area most needing relaxation and rejuvenation.

The quality of the Thai massage you receive may vary widely, even in Thailand. Some therapists have had only a week or two of training and see themselves as giving little more than a half-hour Thai body rub to tourists sunning themselves on the lovely Thai beaches. Then again, you may find an old master with 40 years' experience, who is capable of creating magic.

Unlike most Western forms of massage, Thai massage is per-formed at floor level on a mat. This allows the therapist to skil-fully use his (her) body weight to apply the precise amount of pressure required for each tech-nique. It would be difficult, if not impossible, to perform the

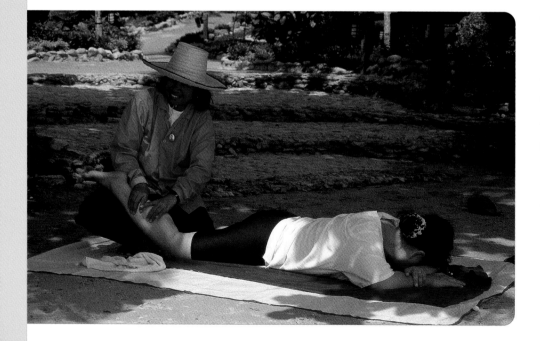

Left Holidaymakers in Thailand often avail themselves of the massage sessions offered on the beach.

THERAPIST–CLIENT TRUST

majority of Thai massage techniques using a massage table. Both client and therapist are fully dressed but usually barefoot. This is one advantage of Thai massage: it eliminates some of the issues associated with giving a massage to an undressed client. A sense of relaxation and trust between client and therapist is built up more easily.

At the start of a massage session, the therapist focuses inwardly, hands held in prayer position (or *namaste*, according to Eastern tradition), as if to ask for assistance or blessing, depending on his personal belief system.

Before you give your first massage, your client should fill out a form, providing personal informa- tion. This should include particulars such as name, address, phone numbers, the client's age and med- ical history, including medications he/she may be taking. Any medical problems should be discussed briefly before the session begins. An indemnity form might also be a good idea. Consult with your lawyer as to having such forms drawn up.

During the massage, the client should be encour- aged to provide feedback as regards any pain or discomfort that might be experienced. In massaging a client, you are entering into a relationship, albeit a very specific and limited one. As in any relation- ship, you need to get to know one another. The client needs to learn to relax, to trust the therapist and to provide accurate feedback. The therapist needs to become used to the body of the client and work around any medical problems that have been discussed and any specific patterns of tension that tend to be habitual.

Some of the techniques used work directly on the *sen* — the energy lines. Others, such as the stretching techniques, affect the energy flow through the *sen* in a more subtle, indirect way. Ultimately, each single technique is aimed at harmonizing or

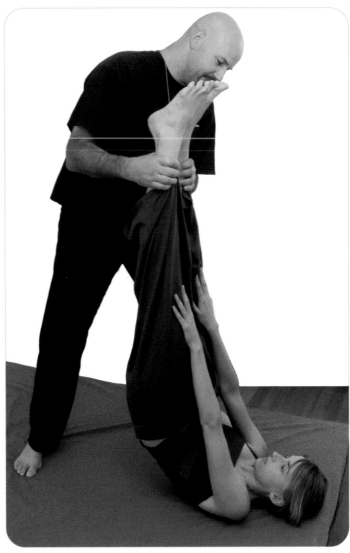

promoting energy flow through the *sen*. The therapist can develop his awareness of this flow of energy by practising continuously and widening his experience with a variety of clients and through exposure to auxiliary practices such as tai chi chuan and meditation.

Above Clients will have varying degrees of suppleness; therefore client–practitioner feedback is crucial during any session.

The basic principles

In starting Thai massage, the apprentice therapist needs to first learn a variety of steps before applying the actual techniques:

* each technique has a set position in which the client is lying or sitting;

* there is a contact point (or points) on the client's body at which the therapist initiates the technique;

* the therapist needs to consider the position of his or her body relative to the client's, and relative to gravity;

* the therapist needs to focus on the movement specific to the technique itself;

* finally, there is the movement from one technique to the next.

Properly executed, a good Thai massage thus becomes a smooth, rhythmic movement sequence, which may remind an onlooker of a slow dance or the execution of a flowing yoga sequence or tai chi routine. It should have that same meditative, gentle quality to it.

The therapist should execute every technique with awareness, both of himself and his client. Self-awareness should include awareness of your posture, your breathing, the amount of pressure you are exerting, and the direction in which it is being exerted. You should also focus on being mentally fully present in the massage rather than daydreaming.

Awareness of your client should include his or her level of muscular tension, energy flow, depth and regularity of breathing, and any sign of discomfort showing on her face.

The rhythm of the massage may be dictated by the client's energy flow, patterns of tension and breathing, but it is physically implemented by the therapist through rhythmical, repetitive weight shifting within a posture, or from one posture to the next.

In giving a Thai massage, and this applies to many other similar practices, true mastery may be described as achieving one's goal with apparent effortlessness, using only exactly that amount of energy required to complete the given task. Using leverage and body weight correctly and being able to transition from one technique to the next without much muscular strain is the benchmark of excellence in performing this form of massage skilfully.

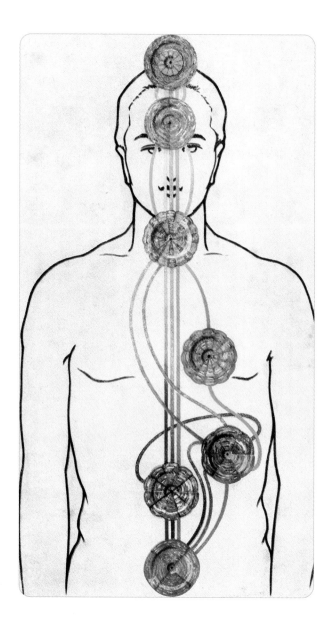

Above **The chakras, or energy centres, are linked by *nadis*, or meridians (energy pathways). Work done on or over these points is believed to promote harmony and balance within the body.**

THE THERAPIST'S RESPONSIBILITIES

One of the prerequisites of a good massage is that the therapist is centred, balanced and confident, both physically and mentally. He or she should not only be able to competently execute the massage techniques but should also put in a certain amount of personal preparation in advance.

In the case of most aspiring massage therapists, sensitivity, open awareness and an attitude of compassion and loving kindness have to be worked at. There is a vast array of meditation methods, visualizations, exercises and training techniques that can help the development of acute self-awareness, and a corresponding awareness of the client, and the relationship between yourself and your client.

Role of meditation

Meditation is often (incorrectly) perceived as something unfathomable and deeply esoteric. For our purposes here, it simply means a conscious and consistent method of focusing on your awareness. It can be an awareness of breathing, posture, movement, or patterns of muscular tension or mental activity.

Breath meditation

One of the simplest and most beneficial meditative practices is breath awareness. This can be done while kneeling or sitting on the floor in a cross-legged position or while sitting on a chair. Kneeling would be the best, as it most closely approximates the position you're in while giving the massage.

Sit quietly and as upright as possible. Gently close your eyes. Rest your hands or forearms on your thighs, palms down or up, whichever is more comfortable. Focus your awareness inward, disregarding any sounds of, say, a clock ticking, the neighbour's hi-fi or the traffic outside. Put the tip of your tongue on the

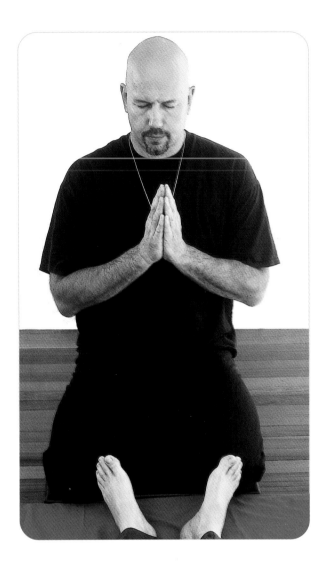

roof of your mouth. Breathe in and out through your nose only. Feel the air as it enters and exits your nostrils. Sense it as it travels down your windpipe and into your lungs. Feel the muscles of your ribcage and abdominal area reacting to the flow of the breath. Become aware of how, as you relax into the practice, your rate of breathing slows down and your breath becomes deeper and deeper. Never force the breath! Just be aware of what is happening, without any conscious interference on your part. Allow the slowing, deepening process but let this happen on its own. The slower it becomes, the more heightened your awareness of finer sensations.

Above right **Before beginning, the therapist should take a quiet moment to centre himself and focus his mind on the session.**

MEDITATION ON MOVEMENT

From the kneeling position, rise up until your thighs are perpendicular to the floor. Shift your weight onto one leg so that it is evenly distributed along the whole of the shin and the instep. Now pick up the leg that is not bearing any weight on it and step forward into one of the more characteristic stances of Thai massage (the thigh and lower leg forming a right angle). Start shifting the weight of your torso and legs forward and backward, in a coherent, unified manner. This movement pattern is used extensively in Thai massage.

Sense what the movement feels like. Which muscles are tense, which are relaxed; how does this change as you move? Are you able to keep your trunk upright or are you inadvertently leaning forward or back? Experiment with what it feels like if your trunk is perpendicular to the floor, then if you are leaning forward. While giving a Thai massage it is not always possible to keep the trunk at right angles to the floor. How do you do so without quickly becoming tired? Once you have played with this — and playful experimentation is always better than plodding seriousness as it's more fun and generates less unnecessary tension — start bringing an awareness of your breath into the practice.

You'll have been breathing all the time, but while your awareness was on the movement you were probably not even aware of your breath. With this renewed awareness, feel what happens as you rock forward and back. When is it best to breathe in? Breathe out? How can you use the slowness of the breath to make the physical movement more relaxed and efficient? Once again, there is no point trying to force anything; simply become more aware of what you are doing and how you are doing it. Remember that this is a process. You are not unaware at one moment and aware the next. You slowly become more aware as you practise more.

Below The intake and outtake of the breath can be co-ordinated with a massage stretch routine to enhance muscular relaxation.

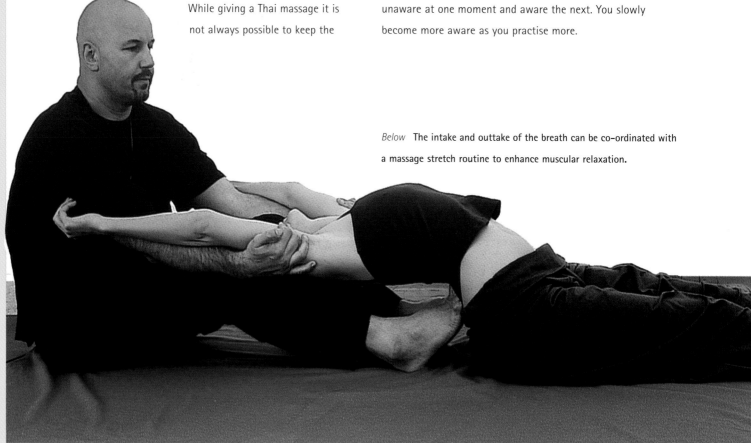

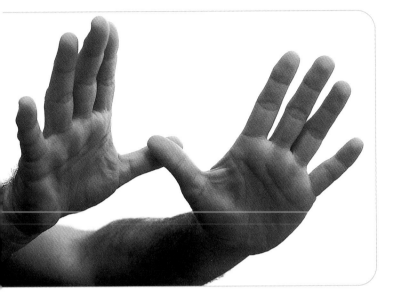

Energy awareness

Once again, sit cross-legged on the floor or kneel. Become
aware of your breathing. Allow it to become deeper and slower.
Feel yourself relax as it does so. Now lift up your hands, holding them in front of your solar plexus as if you were holding an
imaginary soccer ball. The palms are facing each other. Slowly
bring the palms closer together. Sense at what point the air
between the palms starts to feel different. If you are relaxed
and open enough there comes a point at which you perceive a
difference. When this happens and how strong the sensation is
varies greatly from person to person. You may even feel a large
difference when you do this from day to day, depending on
your stress levels, state of health and the ability to open up
your awareness.

The feeling of increasing density between your palms can be
described in a number of ways. It could feel as if you're
squeezing a party balloon; the closer your hands get to each
other, the more resistance you feel. If you initially have problems with feeling anything at all, it may help to use visualizations. The feeling of energy in your palms is often first felt as a
sensation of warmth. You can encourage the process by imag-
ining such warmth. In the Chinese medical and martial traditions it is said, the 'i' leads the 'chi' — meaning that the mind-
intent, or what one chooses to focus one's mind on, will lead or
encourage the energy flow.

To make use of this concept, imagine you are holding a balloon filled with warm water between your hands. Now feel
how the warmth slowly flows from the water into your hands.
Alternatively, you can imagine you're holding warm coals in
your hands. The specific nature of the image is of secondary
importance. You can use whatever makes sense to you and
produces the desired result. What does matter is that you
imagine it strongly. If you do so, you should feel warmth in
your palms and from there on it should be easy to start feeling
the connection between the two palms.

Once you have achieved this, start playing with the awareness. Attempt to feel how the density increases as your palms
come closer together. Try to still feel the energy connection as
you move your palms further and further apart. What happens
if you remove one hand? What happens if you keep the distance between both palms constant but start moving the imaginary ball (still between your hands) around yourself in various
patterns? As you do so, remain aware of both your breathing
and your posture.

These basic explorations of your ability to remain aware of
your breath, posture, movement and energy will all positively
affect your ability to give a good Thai massage. Awareness is
limitless; there is no end to the depth to which it can be
refined. Should you find these exercises interesting and pro-
ductive, you might want to expand your practice by attending
classes on meditation, energy work, yoga or tai chi chuan.

Playing with the breath

While it's easy to say that the therapist should be as fully
aware of himself and his client as possible, gaining awareness
is an ongoing process, and what you can achieve may fluctuate
from moment to moment. Breathing is so central to all movement and all experience that awareness of it is crucial.
Fortunately this is not very difficult to develop. Blood circulation, for instance, is equally central but much more difficult to
become directly aware of.

YOUR POSTURE

Initially, become aware of your own breathing. Then become aware of your client's breathing. Then experiment with how the one can be co-ordinated with the other. Is it better for you to breathe in as he (she) breathes out or should you breathe out at the same time? Does the massage feel different to you or to your client when you synchronize the breathing? How does it help when you ask your client to breathe out during the more strenuous parts of a stretching technique?

When focusing on your posture or how you hold and use your body, a little experimentation quickly shows that there is a right and a wrong way to give a Thai massage. Done correctly, the back is held straight but not rigid, the arms are held straight, and shoulders kept relaxed and not hunched up. By achieving the correct posture, the therapist ensures that all the pressure he wants to exert in a given technique is produced by an interaction of body weight, leverage and gravity.

Since this involves a minimum of muscular tension, the therapist can give several massages in a row without becoming tired. Good posture and body usage also means that you can consciously control the exerted pressure and vary it by whatever minuscule amount you desire. Finally, since the hands and arms of the therapist are acting as sensors, if there is tension in the arms or shoulders, this will minimize the feedback the therapist receives from the client's body.

Alexander technique

Instead of trying to establish the precise angle of your body for every technique, which may vary according to the position of the client and the nature of the technique itself, it is more efficient to educate yourself in correct posture as it pertains to any situation. A good way to do this is to study the Alexander technique, named after its creator, FM Alexander.

This technique primarily creates an awareness of the relationship of the head to the neck and torso. While there is no forced specific exertion to achieve an external, perfect postural form, it promotes an ongoing awareness and a gentle self-

direction. Most of all, you learn to remind yourself to hold the head forward and up and to feel the torso lengthening and broadening. On paper this may sound fairly simple, but as anyone who has ever studied the Alexander technique extensively will tell you, it takes a lot of time, energy and conscious self-direction to achieve such awareness.

Once you have succeeded in doing this, it becomes unnecessary to worry about the postural specifics of any of the massage techniques as you'll automatically be executing them with the correct use of your body.

Below Shivago Komarpaj, a respected Ayurvedic practitioner from India, was in fact the founding father of Thai massage and the ancient Indian healing tradition of Thai Ayurveda.

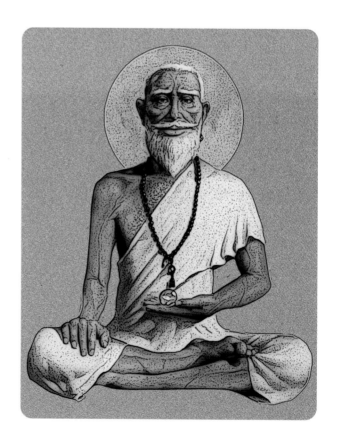

LIMITATIONS AND CONTRAINDICATIONS

Do bear in mind that Thai massage — and any other form of massage, for that matter — is not a panacea. If, as a trainee or fulltime therapist, you suspect that the client may have medical problems, it is your duty to recommend that the client see a doctor as soon as possible. If, as a therapist, you have the slightest doubt about the appropriateness of giving a massage, you should refrain from doing so.

There are a variety of conditions for which Thai massage or some of its techniques are contraindicated. The major ones are as follows:

* **High blood pressure**: In this case, avoid massaging the abdominal area. Also, avoid postures in which both legs are raised.
* **Varicose veins, phlebitis (inflammation of a vein) or thrombosis**: Never exert direct pressure on veins or areas thus affected.
* **Circulatory system–related problems**: If you are told or suspect that there are any such problems (e.g. arteriosclerosis), avoid postures that might increase pressure in the arteries.
* **Skin disorders**: Do not massage these areas; find out from the client whether the condition is communicable (in other words, capable of being passed on readily).
* **Bruises, fractures or swelling**: Do not massage on top of affected areas.
* **Spine/skeletal structure**: Do not massage directly over bone or on top of the spine itself.
* **Arthritis or degeneration in the joint**: If you can feel that there is such a condition, do not apply range-of-motion stretches to a joint.
* **Pregnant women**: Do not force stretches to their extreme. Avoid inverted postures. Avoid direct pressure to the web of the thumb. After the third or fourth month of pregnancy, it is recommended to use the side-lying and seated positions only.

In many ways a good general guideline is that the older the client, the gentler the massage should be.

Note: Before starting with a massage on a new client, you should be informed as to his or her medical history and state of health. He should fill out a medical ailments form (see p122-3) and you then need to discuss his general health with him. If you have any doubts at all, it's recommended that you err on the side of caution. Ask your client to consult with his or her doctor as to whether Thai massage is a good idea. When Thai massage is used to treat a condition it was not intended for, it might actually prove to be harmful.

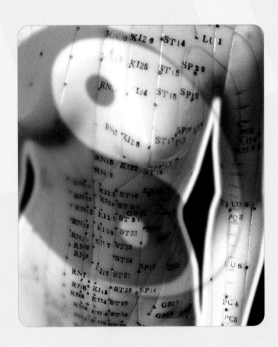

Right **Acupuncture points used in traditional Chinese medicine are marked up on a mannequin for use in the teaching of students.**

USEFUL TIPS

Massage vs. bodywork

Since the spectrum of possible treatments has become so broad in recent years, many practitioners now refer to what they are doing as 'bodywork', a term previously used only in the motor vehicle repair business!

The ethics of touch

Thai massage does not have any of the potential ethical problems of other forms of massage (e.g. client nudity). There is a fair amount of contact with the client's body, though, so care should be taken to explain the need for certain positions.

Keeping the client warm

A good massage should have a relaxing effect on the client; if she feels cold, she will automatically tense up. It is therefore essential to have the room temperature at a suitable level. In Thailand, due to the tropical weather, this is not an issue.

To talk or not to talk

Some clients prefer to experience their massage silently, others cannot stop talking. It is best to follow the client's lead in this. Since a Thai massage is a process of communication, there are no rules for this beyond that of making the client feel at ease.

The use of music

Music may be soothing and helpful in relaxing both client and therapist. To create a pleasant atmosphere the volume should be kept fairly low. There is a great variety of music available, some of it specifically composed for massage treatments.

Sensitivity training

One of the most effective ways to train manual sensitivity, that is, to teach your fingers and hands to 'hear' what the client's body is 'communicating', is to practise the various massage techniques with your eyes closed.

Visualization

To enhance a client's ability to relax, you could ask him to close his eyes and imagine himself in a beautiful natural setting, such as a tropical island beach or a mountain meadow beside a stream or lake. This works especially well with carefully selected music.

Therapist's feedback

Since the massage is a communicative process, feedback helps the process for the client. Pointing out areas of greater tension may not necessarily provide her with any new information but may help establish confidence in your sensitivity and ability as a therapist. Advice as to possible stretching or breathing techniques she may use to prevent the recurrence of certain problems will help to carry forward the beneficial effects of your work into your client's daily life.

Client's feedback

In turn, ask your client to give you feedback. This lets you know when you are applying too much pressure or causing extreme pain or pleasure. It also draws your client into the process and empowers her.

Body support

Since spinal curvature and posture may vary from client to client, it is useful to have a selection of cushions, bolsters and pillows of varying sizes and thickness to support the head or to put underneath the client's abdominal area when he is lying chest down on the mat. The more supported the body feels, the easier it is for the client to relax.

Art vs. science

Massage is an art, not a science. If it were a science, this would imply that one could consistently achieve the same results using the same methods in treating the same problems. In reality, clients differ, their problems differ and what works for them is

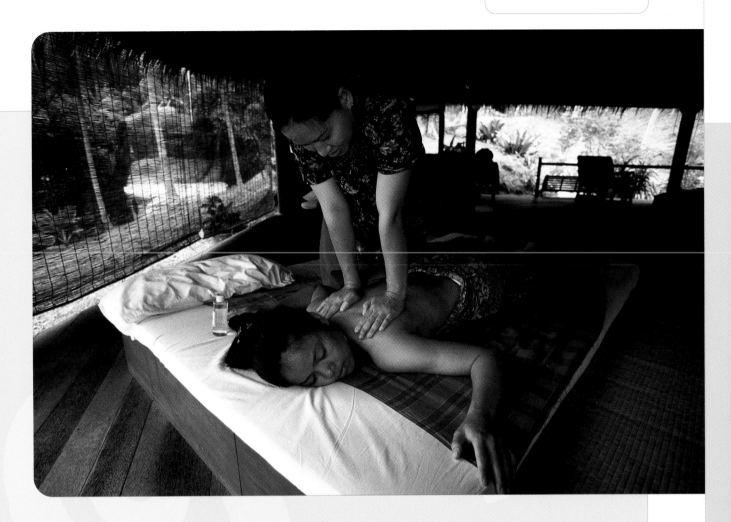

also different. Intuitive sensitivity belongs in the province of art, which is a key component in giving a good massage.

Educating the client

If a client comes to you regularly, this becomes an opportunity to educate him with regard to his body. You can point out patterns of tension and how these patterns tend to reappear between treatments. You can teach him some basic stretching, breathing and relaxation techniques. In this way, he can learn to take some responsibility for his own healing and growth.

Above **A Thai massage practitioner applies palm presses to the upper back of a client, inducing a state of extreme relaxation.**

Energy levels

Experiments with natural healers have shown that the healer's energy levels may significantly affect those of the client. In other words, if the therapist is feeling sick, irritable or de-energized, this is likely to be transferred to the client on a subtle level. It is therefore important to work on your own energy level by means of breathing exercises, visualizations, yoga, tai chi chuan, and similar practices.

Studying anatomy

Although some massage associations stipulate certification on anatomy for membership purposes, historically speaking Thai massage was developed without any knowledge of anatomical structures. Its preferred focus is the intuitive approach.

THE SEN LINES

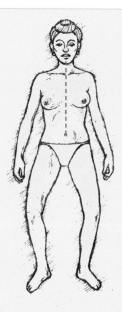

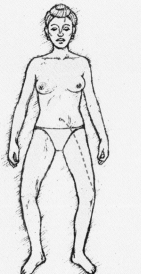

Sen Sumana starts at tip of tongue, runs down throat and chest into solar plexus

Sen Ittha starts at left nostril, runs over scalp, down throat and neck, down back (line 1), over left buttocks and becomes line 3 on back of leg. Crosses front of knee and becomes line 1 on inside thigh, runs up front leg to left side of navel.

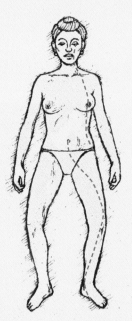

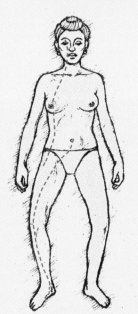

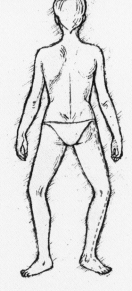

Sen Sahatsarangsi starts in left eye, runs down throat, left side of chest and abdomen, and around to outside of leg. Becomes line 1 on back leg, runs into foot, around instep, then up inside leg (line 1). Crosses groin and stops just below navel.

Sen Thawari begins in the right eye, and follows identical pathway to Sen Sahatsarangsi but on the right side.

THE SEN LINES

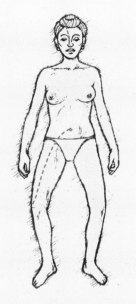

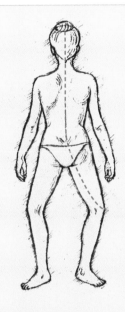

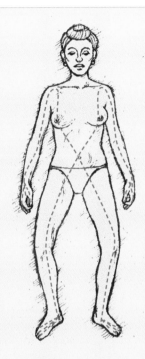

Sen Kalathari starts at navel, branches into two upper pathways, each one running through abdomen, chest, up to shoulder and down central inner arm to palm. From here branches to the tips of each finger. Lower branched pathways run across inner groin, become line 2 down inside leg to foot, then branch to each toe.

Sen Pingkhala is identical to Sen Ittha, but runs along the right side of the body.

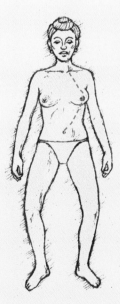

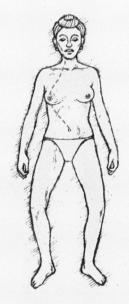

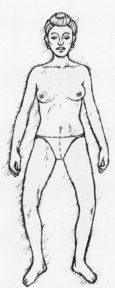

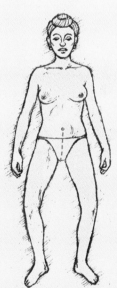

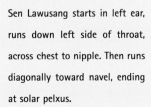

Sen Lawusang starts in left ear, runs down left side of throat, across chest to nipple. Then runs diagonally toward navel, ending at solar pelxus.

Sen Ulangka starts in right ear and follows same path as Sen Lawusang but on the right side.

Sen Nanthakrawat comprises two pathways. The first runs from navel through urethra, ending at urine passageway. The second runs from navel through colon to anus.

Sen Khitchanna runs from navel to penis (men); from navel through uterus into vagina (women).

Part Two
The massage session

THERE ARE FOUR BASIC BODY POSITIONS that apply in Thai massage. Traditionally, you start with the client lying flat on the back. From there you proceed to the side-lying position, then the client turns over onto his or her stomach, and this is followed by sitting upright in a cross-legged position. To close off the massage, the client once again lies supine while the therapist works on the shoulders, neck, head and face.

If the therapist is giving an abbreviated massage, or it takes place in an office environment, or time is limited, he can start with the seated position. This allows him to immediately access the shoulders and the neck – areas that most commonly react to stress by tightening up. Since Thai massage is based on harmonizing the energy flow of the whole body via the energy lines, it often happens that the client will experience strong sensations, such as feelings of warmth, energy circulation or a release in the upper body while the therapist is working on the energy lines of the legs. If, in accordance with Eastern philosophy, you see the body as an interconnected matrix of energy, then it follows that work done on a specific part may help another part.

A client looking for a general treatment aimed at relaxation and overall balancing of the body's energy will be treated differently from someone coming in with a specific complaint such as a backache.

PREPARATION

Thai massage is given in a spirit of loving kindness, and with an open and aware attitude, so it is common for the therapist to say a meditative prayer before starting with the massage itself. This serves to clear the mind and to transition from the reality of everyday life to the meditative flow of the massage. Traditionally, it is a prayer to the memory of the founder of Thai massage, Shivago Komarpaj, but it can take any form you are comfortable with, as long as it achieves its calming purpose. After the prayer, circle the hands together quietly to generate warmth and to initiate the energy flow and stimulate your awareness of your hands, then start by massaging the feet.

Right The client takes up a supine position in both the beginning and final phases of a Thai massage.

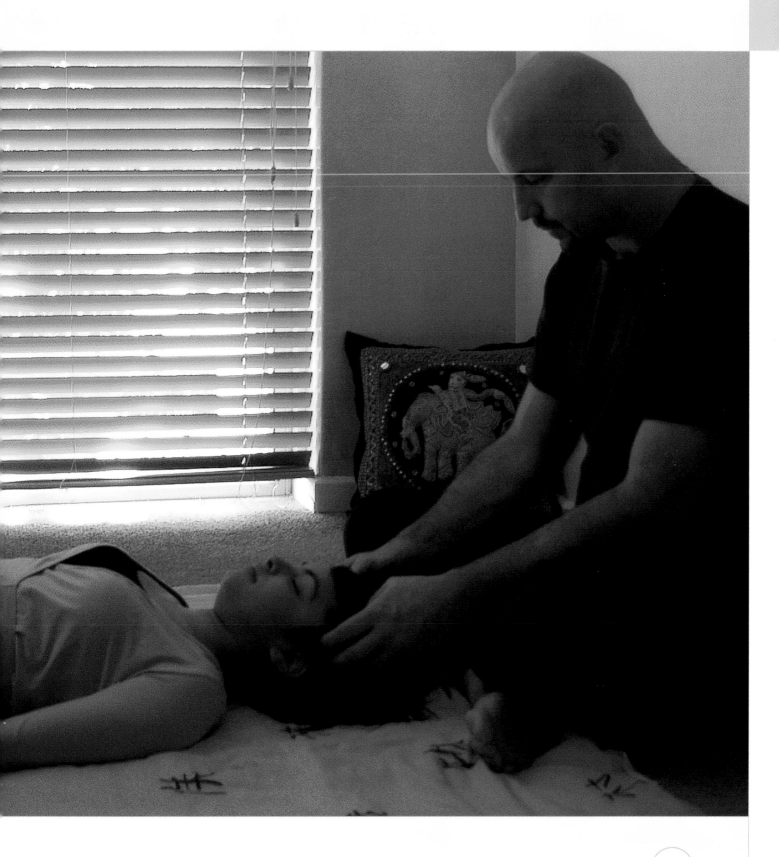

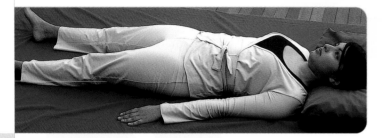

Lying on the back

PROCEDURES 1-41

Starting with the feet and ankles has several advantages. It serves as a warm-up before proceeding to the more specific problem areas such as the legs, back, shoulders or neck. Also, it feels fairly noninvasive. If the practitioner were to start, for instance, with the abdominal area, the intensity of sensation might be such that it would be difficult for the client to allow him- or herself to slip into the receptive and relaxed state best suited to receiving the treatment. Keeping in mind the length of time needed for the massage and any areas of the body that might need specific attention, the therapist has to establish a rhythm and pace that will be maintained for the duration of the whole massage.

Although working the feet first may serve as a type of warm-up for massaging the rest of the body, it must be remembered that, in terms of the interconnectedness of the energy lines, the feet are every bit as important as any other part of the body. With reflexology, for example, the reflexologist believes that different areas of the foot are representative of corresponding areas in the body, and that healing can be stimulated by concentrating on the feet. You should therefore avoid rushing through your working of the feet, and even the legs, to get to more 'important' areas such as the back and shoulders. Every area of the body is interconnected and it is important that the flow you establish at the beginning of the massage is maintained throughout.

When working the energy lines of the legs, be very aware of feedback. Certain areas, especially on the outer thigh, may be very sensitive to pressure. After you have given massages for a while, you will intuitively feel what the correct rhythm and pace should be for a particular treatment. If you follow your intuition and are aware of your breathing, posture and movement and that of the client, then the natural, flowing quality of Thai massage will come

into play. To both yourself and your client the massage will then feel like a beautiful dance and both of you will feel more energized at the end of it than you were before you started.

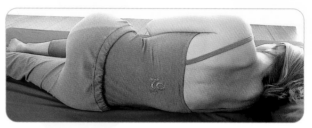

Lying on the side

PROCEDURES 42—51

In the side-lying position, ensure that your client's lower leg is fully extended and that the upper leg is bent at a 90-degree angle. Using cushions, see to it that the head is fully supported. Should the client feel any strain in the neck or shoulders because of having to support some of the weight of her head, this will make the position extremely uncomfortable for her. It may also be advisable to use a pillow to support the bent leg at the knee.

The side-lying position is especially valuable for pregnant women; some of the other positions may become uncomfortable or completely impossible during the course of pregnancy. It is the position in which many clients are often at their most relaxed; some may even fall asleep during the massage.

In this position you have good access to the client's back, hip area and the energy lines of the legs. In terms of the positioning of your own body, you must take into consideration that some of the areas you are now working on are much more elevated than they were when the client was lying on her back. You need to change your own stance and posture accordingly, otherwise you may find yourself experiencing tension and discomfort through your bad posture. This in turn takes your awareness away from the client as you'll focus on what you're feeling rather than on what the client is feeling. Consequently, the quality of the massage will suffer.

Even though you may have fully supported your client and made sure she was correctly aligned, it's quite possible that she will move while being massaged. Working with pressure on the client's back may cause the bent knee to slide forward, possibly leading to her spine being misaligned in her side-lying posture. You need to be aware of this and ready to reposition your client's body when necessary. This is where the supporting pillow under the knee may come in useful, functioning as a brace against the surface of the massage mat. Without it the client may repeatedly move out of alignment or, alternatively, need to use muscular tension in an attempt to maintain alignment on her own.

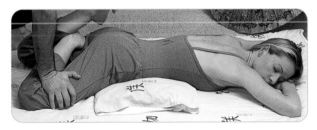

Lying on the stomach

PROCEDURES	52–69

A high percentage of people opting for a massage come to the therapist's mat because of back pain or back problems. The back is accessible in both the side-lying and seated position, but the best position for in-depth massage of the back is with the client lying on his stomach. The counterpressure of the floor and the mat allows the therapist to exert as much pressure as is comfortable for the client, to really work the energy lines and the muscular structure of the back in a deep and intense way.

The client may choose to lie with the face down, in which case he will either support his own forehead with his forearms or use a cushion for this purpose. Without either of these the nose is pressed into the mat and it becomes difficult to breathe freely. Should the client prefer to turn his head to the side, it is advisable to ask him occasionally to switch sides to avoid stiffness in the neck. It is usually also very helpful to put a pillow under the client's abdomen to support and straighten out the lower back. Should the client have very stiff ankles, it is good to put small pillows under each foot.

Seated upright

PROCEDURES	70–88

Here the client sits upright with her legs crossed. She can keep her hands in her lap or at her sides. At this stage of the massage, the client should be in a fairly relaxed, though energized, state from the work done in the previous three positions.

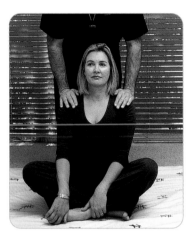

Techniques you use for working on the client's back in this position are essentially to 'finish off' the work done on the back in the previous positions. The importance of the upright posture lies in the ease of access to the shoulder area, especially the trapezius muscle and surrounding area; it also allows you to begin working with the client's neck. This work done on the neck is then finished off when the client again lies on her back in the concluding phase of the massage.

Some clients, especially those experiencing pain in their lower back, may find this position uncomfortable. In this case, you will minimize the time spent here or avoid it altogether. As a result of the great variety of techniques available in the field of Thai massage, it's possible to access all areas and energy lines despite having to leave out perhaps one of the basic positions.

Although the work done on the neck in this position does contribute to relaxation and the flow of energy, it will not have as deep an effect as when the client is lying on her back. This is simply because the head is heavy, and a good deal of muscular tension is necessary to prevent it from dropping forward while sitting upright. This tension counteracts the deep relaxation the client experiences lying on her back.

Lying on the back

TRADITIONALLY, THAI MASSAGE ALWAYS BEGINS with the client lying on his or her back. This position allows a much higher degree of relaxation as no postural muscles have to be engaged to maintain an upright position. It also allows the therapist the best access to all parts of the client's legs. In cultural and economic terms, Thailand differs from the European or American city environment where back and shoulder problems are prevalent as a result of mainly deskbound professions. In Thailand, most of the clientele are likely to suffer from aches and pains in the legs due to being on their feet all day — working in the fields, in construction or as salespeople on the shop floor. In Thailand, work on the legs may take up as much as half the time allocated for the whole massage.

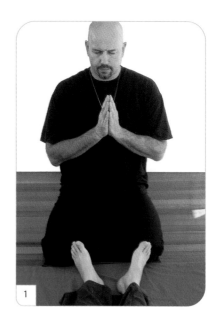

The client lies on her back with the therapist kneeling at her feet.

1 Before you begin, compose yourself by saying a short prayer or doing a brief meditation. The massage is to be given in a spirit of 'loving kindness' — as the Thais put it, 'Warm heart, warm hands'. Rub your hands together to create warmth. Place the client's feet shoulder width apart. You will use the whole of the hand to create pressure, a technique called the 'palm press'.

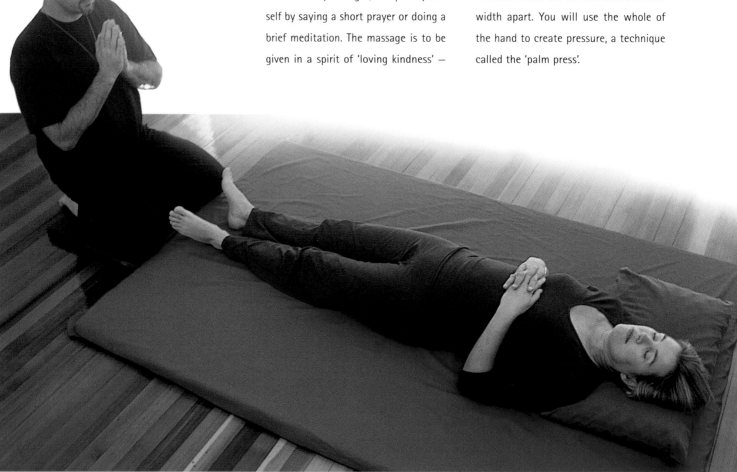

WARMING UP FEET AND LEGS

1 Place your hands on the feet, just below the ankles. Maintaining straight arms, allow your body weight to press down while you gently stretch the feet outward. Release and move your hands slightly toward the toes. Once again apply pressure. Do this three or four times until you have covered the entire top part of the foot to the toes. Conclude by firmly pressing on the heels.

2 Now, rocking your body weight from side to side, use alternating palm presses to once again work both feet, then, maintaining this alternating rhythm, walk your hands up the client's calves. As in all Thai massage, avoid direct pressure on bone, in this case the tibia.

3 4 When you reach the client's knees, gently cup the kneecap with your palms and make three or four little circular movements. Continue with alternating palm presses up the client's thigh until you reach the point where the legs meet the groin (inguinal crease). While working your way up the thigh, make sure you're not pressing so hard that you 'roll' the muscle over the bone beneath.

Therapist's posture

By keeping your posture aligned and upright and the arms locked out straight, you can control very precisely the amount of pressure you exert on the client. You also eliminate unnecessary tension in your body and can thus sense the client's response far better than if you were massaging using localized muscular tension in your arms only. Spread the pressure over your whole hand. If you concentrate it within the palm only, it may be too penetrating for many clients.

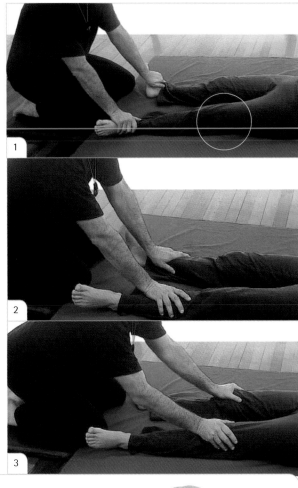

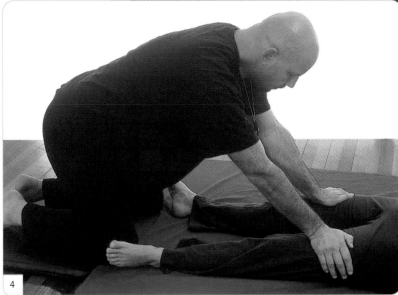

PRESSURE POINTS OF FEET

Once again, with your arms locked out straight, you use carefully applied body weight to create pressure on the sole of the foot. As before, shift your body from side to side, creating a gentle, alternating, rhythmic rocking motion. This time you do not use your palm, though; you concentrate the pressure into a far smaller area by using your thumbs.

Technique

Care has to be taken with the position of the thumb. If your thumb is held too vertical, i.e. almost at a right angle to the sole, the pressure will be too intense and there is a risk of damaging your thumbs over time. Alternatively, if you press with

Right **The six pressure points of the feet. If there is sufficient time, it is enormously beneficial to massage the entire underside of the foot.**

your thumb held almost parallel to the area being worked, you will not generate enough pressure. You need to find a middle path.

1 – 3 Working with both hands, alternately thumb press on the six pressure points indicated, in the given numerical order. Do three circuits. On the first and the third circuit, exert pressure for five seconds on each of the points. On

the second circuit, press firmly for 10 seconds on each point. While pressing, use the rest of your hand to open the client's foot outward. To finish off this technique, do palm presses on both feet.

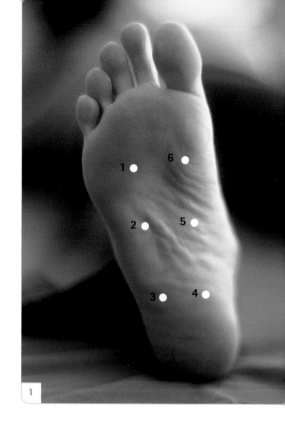

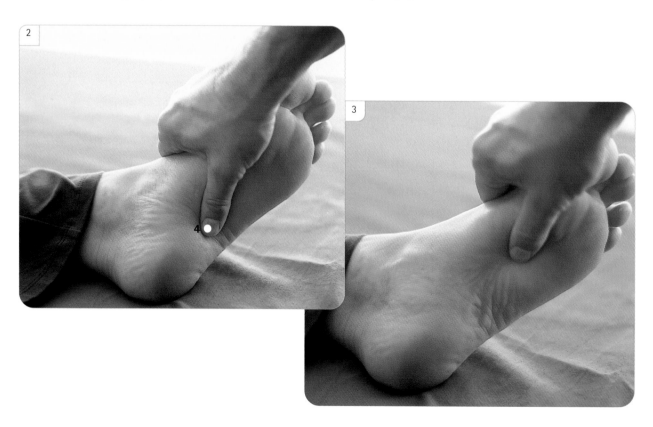

1

2

3

THUMB PRESSES TO ENERGY LINES

[1] [2] Visualize the five energy lines flowing from a point just in from the centre of the heel, each line running through one of the toes. You no longer use an alternating, rocking motion but press both feet simultaneously. Starting with the inner line running to the big toe, work your way up from the heel.

[3]-[5] Thumb press until you reach the ball of the foot, then do small circular rubbing motions with the thumbs, called 'thumb circles'. When you reach the tip of the toe, pinch it gently, then release it and begin working on the next line, starting from the heel area. Finish off with alternating palm presses to the soles of the feet.

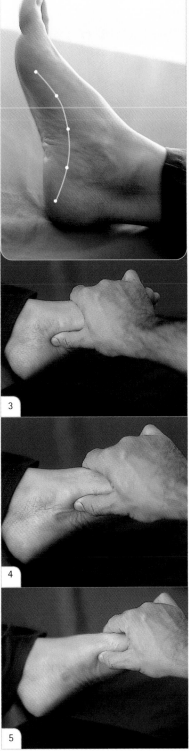

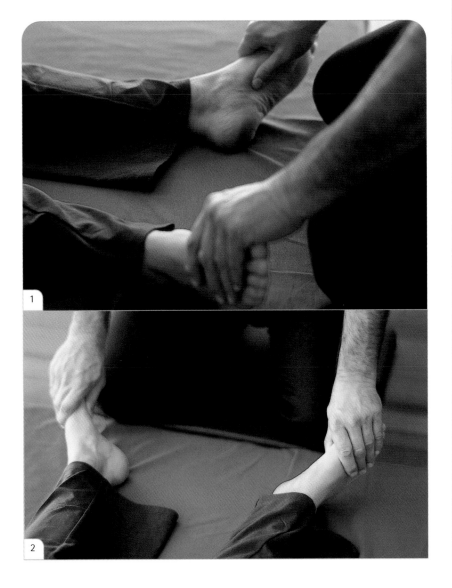

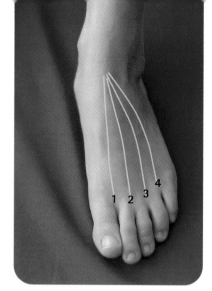

WORKING THE ENERGY LINES OF THE FEET

Turn both of the client's feet upward, so that the big toe is pointing toward the ceiling. If necessary, adjust the position of the client's legs so that they are just a little further apart than the outside of your knees. This is done to ensure that you apply pressure downward with the correct alignment and use of your body weight.

1 Rise from your kneeling position until you are above the client's feet. Now palm press directly downward on the foot just below the ankle, then mid-foot, then over the toes. Thereafter, work backward — i.e. mid-foot and in front of the ankle. When you are palm pressing the toes, do not bend the foot downward. The pressure should still go into the heel.

2 Now work the four energy lines on top of the foot; these start at the hollow at the centre of the ankle joint and run along the grooves between the tendons of the foot. Thumb press the hollow, then do thumb circles all along the first groove, between first and big toe. When you reach the toe, briefly pinch the area between the toes. Then thumb circle the toe, hold it, pinch and pull it gently, and release.

When you reach the little toes, do finger circles, using the fingertips, on the edge of the toes, hold them, then pinch and pull them.

Above The four energy lines along the top of the foot run between the tendons. Gentler pressure is applied to bony areas, with a stronger massage technique between the tendons.

To complete this technique, repeat the palm pressing sequence you used to begin this procedure along the top of the feet.

In many of the techniques, palm presses are used both at the beginning and end of the session to warm up the area to be worked on and as a gentle, repetitious transition between different techniques.

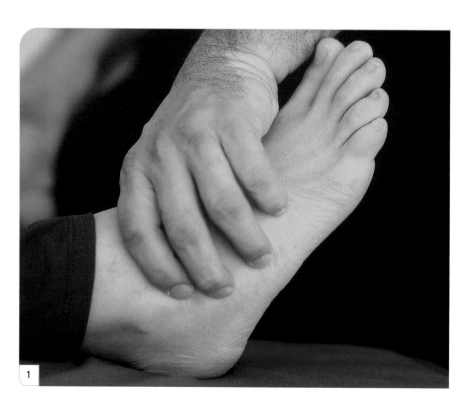

1

ANKLE ROTATION

Sit comfortably in a cross-legged position, straightening one leg slightly to support the leg you're working on (the left leg first for women, right for men).

1 Cup the ankle with one of your hands and cup the front of the foot with the other.

2 – 6 Gently but precisely rotate the foot five times in one direction, five times in the other. According to tradition, you do the left leg (or side) first for women and the right side for men. Circle outward first. If your client is a woman, you circle her left foot in a clockwise direction.

The hand you use to cup the ankle, and thus hold the weight of the client's leg, rests on your thigh to avoid muscular fatigue on your part. Most of the movement comes from the hand you use to cup the toes.

If you find it difficult to create movement around the ankle, you can increase the pressure you're exerting by pushing or pulling in the opposite direction to the hand that's supporting the ankle. If this is still not sufficient, you can use the weight of your upper body to lean into the technique. The more pressure you exert, the more slowly you execute the technique. It is also safer because you have greater control.

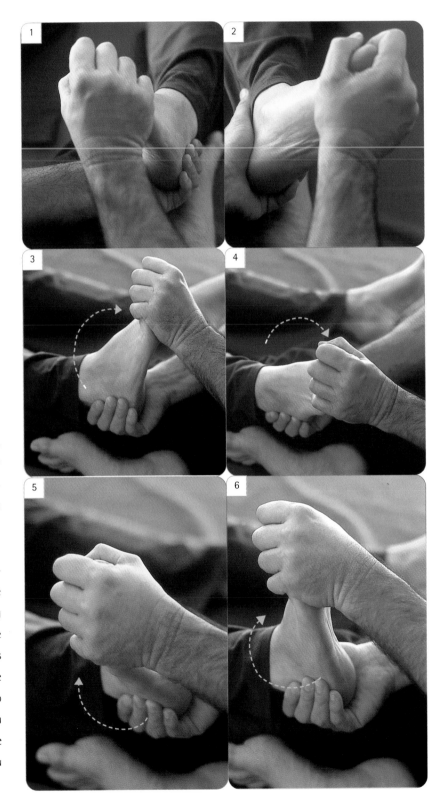

TWISTING OF THE FOOT

Support the client's ankle from underneath with one hand. The first twist is done toward the outer edge of the client's body. So, if your client is a woman, you work with her left foot first, supporting her ankle from underneath with your left hand. Your right palm covers her instep, with your fingers hooking over and around onto the sole of her foot.

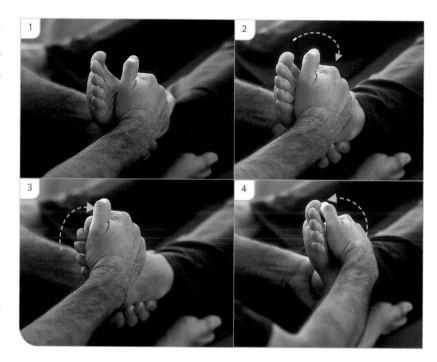

1 For the first twist, start with your hand positioned very close to her ankle. Lean back, thereby using your body weight to give you the leverage required to twist the foot. 2 Then reposition your hand on the middle of her instep and again lean back and twist.

3 Repeat for a third outward twist while holding the toes, then go back the same way you came, 4 twisting once more at mid-instep and once at the ankle.

The twists done at the ankle are done fairly gently, the ones done on the foot are done quite vigorously. At the ankle, all the pressure exerted acts on the ankle directly. At the foot, the very flexible bone structure allows most of the pressure exerted to dissipate before it has an effect on the ankle joint.

5 6 Then change hands, the previously active hand now supporting the ankle from underneath. Using the opposite hand, twist the ankle in the opposite direction. Once again, you move from the outer ankle inward, for a total of five twists.

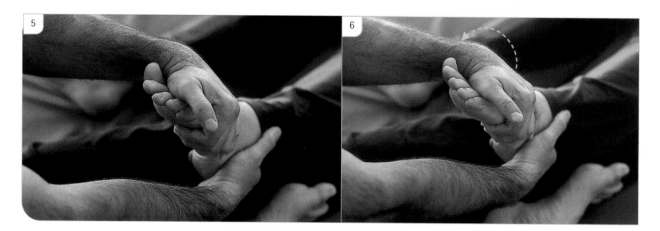

ARCH AND CALF STRETCH

Place the client's heels together or very close to each other. 1 Come up so that you are kneeling on one leg, with your other leg supporting you, foot on the floor, thigh at right angles to your calf. You are thus positioned directly above the client's ankles, enabling you to apply controlled pressure directly downward.

2 Press downward on the feet. Rock your own body forward above the client's ankles as you press down — this makes the technique more flowing and the pressure exerted feel less rigid. First press just below the ankle, next the mid-foot over the instep, then the toes, and back to the mid-foot, and ankle. Each time you palm press, maintain the pressure for five seconds. When your hands are over the arch, press gently. When you press down on the toes, do so firmly.

Then squat with your weight on the balls of both feet and 3 curl your fingers around her toes, 4 clasping them firmly. Rock forward, pressing the heels of your hands into the balls of the toes to stretch the back of the calf as you gently push the feet away from you.

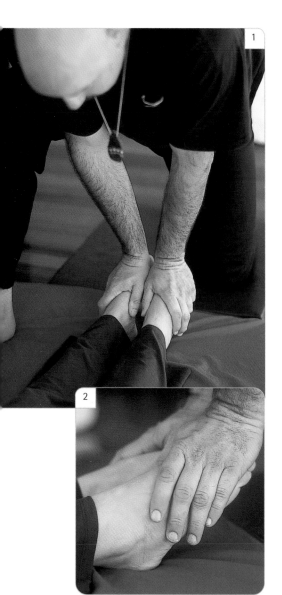

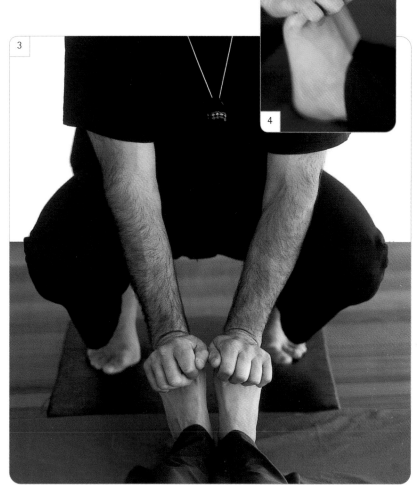

ENERGY LINES ON INNER LEG

The energy lines on the legs are highly important in Thai massage. There are three lines on the inside and three on the outside of each leg. If you are working on a female client, it is traditional to work on the inside of her left leg first (although the photographs show the right leg being worked on). Kneel or half-kneel on the outside of her leg. If you half-kneel, the raised knee should be the one closer to the client's foot.

[1] Begin by stretching the opposite leg from the groin (inguinal fold) to the ankle by means of downward palm presses to both areas. [2] Do a walking palm press — done by shifting your weight from palm to palm as you walk them along the limb — from the ankle to the upper thigh and back down again. Remember, no direct pressure onto bone, so skip over the knee. On reaching the ankle, do an ankle stretch by holding the ankle with one hand and moving the foot with the other one.

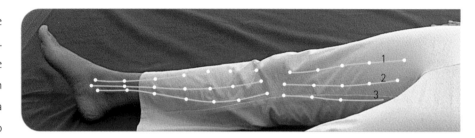

Above **The three energy lines of the inner leg.**

Now use thumb presses on the energy lines of the inner leg. [3] [4] Work the top line first, beginning in the little hollow just underneath the ankle, working your way up the groove between the tibia and the calf muscle.

[5] From the knee, **line 1** runs from the inside edge of the patella (kneecap) to the groin. Do walking thumb presses up line 1 and down again. Use the fleshy part of your thumb, creating a flowing, steady rhythm. Usually you do a thumb press

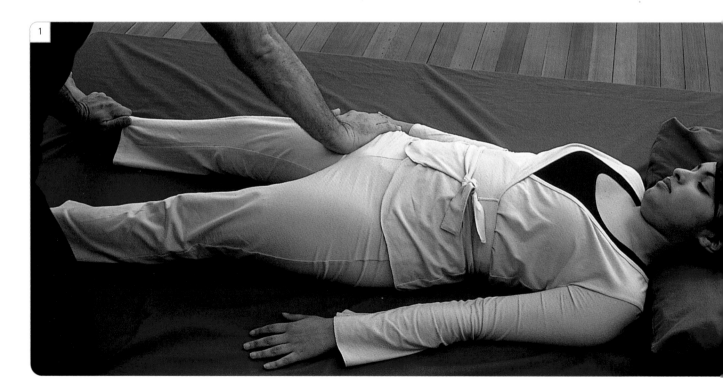

THUMB PRESSES ON INNER LEG

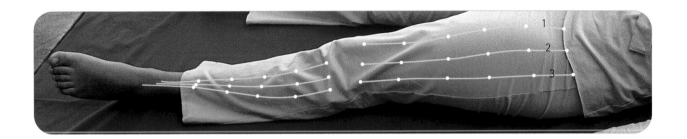

every 5—7.5cm (2—3in). What's important is the slow, rhythmical movement. If you are short of time, instead of doing the same number of presses hurriedly, rather space the presses further apart. Remember to keep your arms extended for the thumb presses so that you are using body weight, not arm muscle. Keep your back straight for the same reason — and to avoid backache.
Line 2 runs along the middle of the calf muscle; it lies about the length of the client's thumb below line 1, on the client's thigh, ending at the pulse spot of the femoral artery.
Line 3 runs from the edge of the Achilles tendon to the tendon behind the knee, from this tendon and along the thigh to the

Above   **The three energy lines of the outer leg.**

groin, about one thumb's length down from line 2. If line 3 is a little difficult to access, use your fingers to push the client's leg over slightly, thereby exposing the line. Execute thumb presses on line 2, then line 3, up each line and down again. After a few months of practice you will develop a feeling for where the energy lines are and you will be able to intuitively feel when you are not on target. Watch the client carefully and ask for feedback, as sensitivity on the lines may vary widely. If the pressure

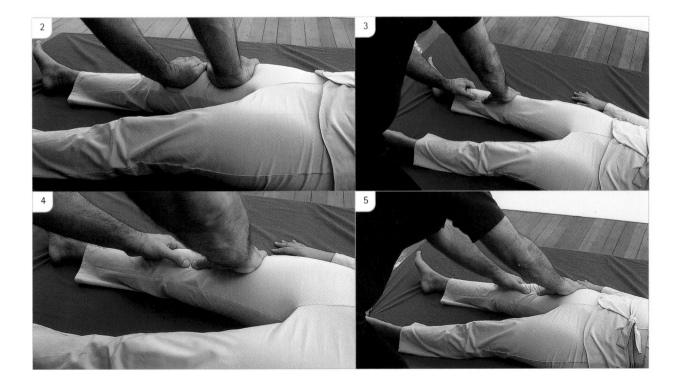

THUMB PRESSES TO OUTER LEG

is too great, the client will tense up. This tension negates the positive effects of the massage. After working all three energy lines, do a palm press walk up and down the inside of the leg, finishing with an ankle stretch.

Now work the energy lines on the outside of the client's other leg (refer to illustrations, pp42–43). First, stretch the outer leg by simultaneously pressing one palm against the outer hip, just below the hip bone, and the other palm against the outer edge of the foot, opposite the instep. Then do alternating palm presses up the outside of the leg and down again, finishing with an ankle stretch. Kneeling on one leg, use the ball of your foot on the other leg (out of the confines of the photograph) to push your client's leg slightly inward to expose the outer energy lines. 1 2 Slowly and rhythmically thumb press your way up the first, uppermost energy line and then down again. Do the same with the second and the 3 third energy line. Once again finish off by palm pressing up and down the outer leg and doing an ankle stretch.

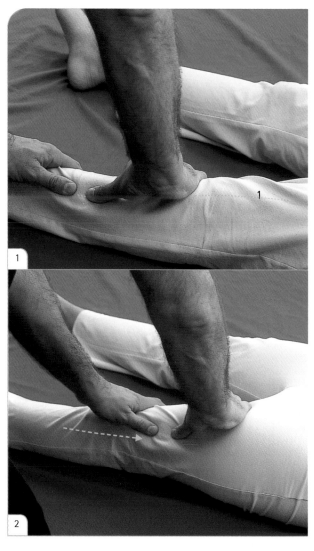

Now switch your position to the outside of the client's other leg and repeat this sequence on the other side.

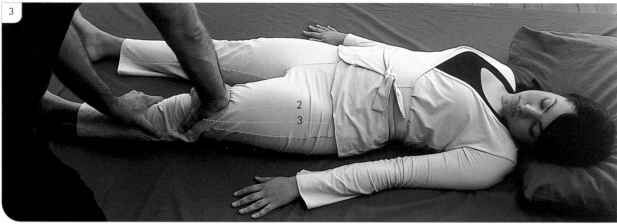

PALM PRESSES ON BENT LEG

Bend your client's leg so that the heel of the bent leg is beside the knee of the other leg. Place one hand above each knee (one bent, one straight) and press downward. Do alternating palm presses moving up each thigh to just below the groin and back to the knee again.

Shift your position so that your body faces the shin of the bent leg. With one palm on the ankle of the bent leg and one just below the knee, walk the palms toward each other in an alternating fashion. When they meet in the middle of the calf, walk them out again. Then position one hand just above the knee and the other just below the groin. Walk the palms in toward each other and out to their starting position again.

1 Starting with one hand on the foot of the bent leg and the other on the thigh just above the knee, walk one palm up the calf, the other palm up the thigh, alternating your palms. Then walk down again.

2 Finally, put both hands on the thigh above the knee in the butterfly position and do simultaneous butterfly palm presses up the thigh to the groin and back down again. Repeat this five times, pressing softly the first time, with medium pressure the second, hard the third, then medium and finally softly again.

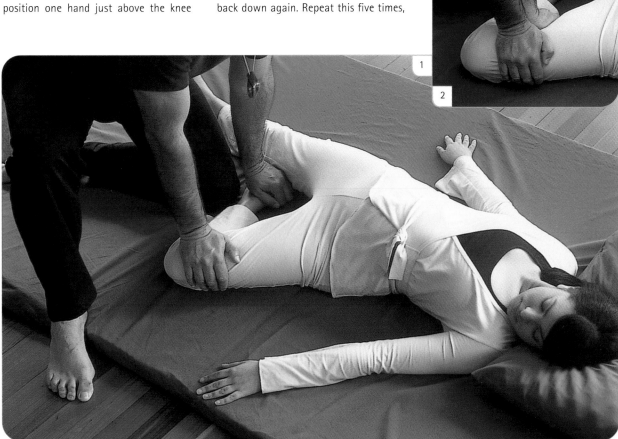

FOOT PRESS TO THIGH

Starting from the bent leg position used in the previous technique, open out the leg and sit between the legs. With each hand, take hold of each of the ankles to support and brace them.

1 With one foot supporting the inner thigh (photo demonstrates left leg), place the sole of your other foot against the back of your client's bent thigh, just inside of the knee. Push and extend your leg, creating medium to strong pressure at the exact moment your leg straightens at the knee. Create counterpressure by pulling back moderately on the ankle of the bent leg. Place your foot at the mid-thigh and repeat, 2 doing the same for the upper thigh, the mid-thigh and back near the knee again.

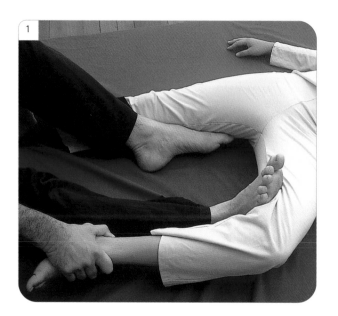

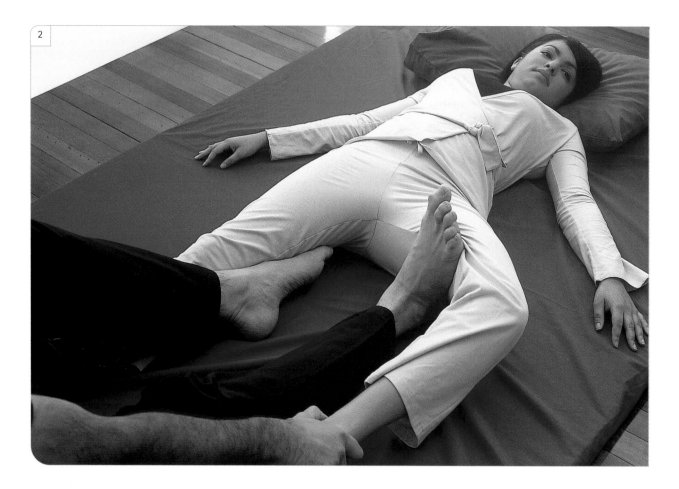

WORKING THE INNER THIGH

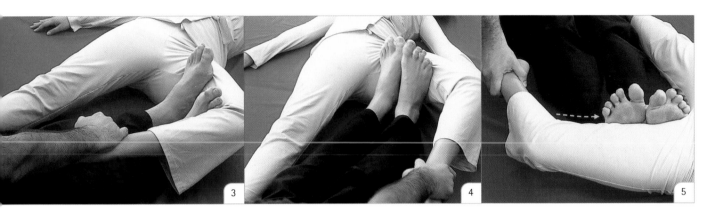

3 | 4 | 5

3 – 5 While holding firmly onto the ankles, use the soles of both feet to walk up and down the inner thigh, from groin to knee, several times. If you do this fairly lightly and rhythmically, it is very relaxing for the client.

6 Now fold one leg inward so that her sole almost touches the inner thigh of her opposite leg. Anchor the bent inner thigh with your foot and use your fingers 7 to 'hook' over the upper thigh muscles and pull them toward you.

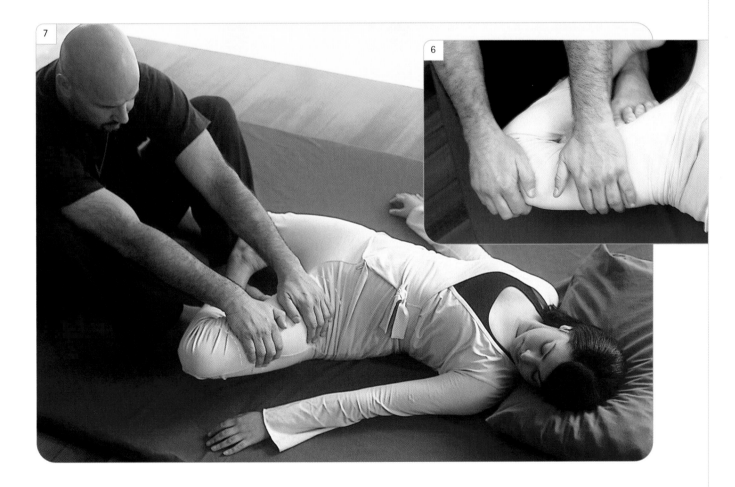

7

6

ENERGY LINES ON THE THIGH

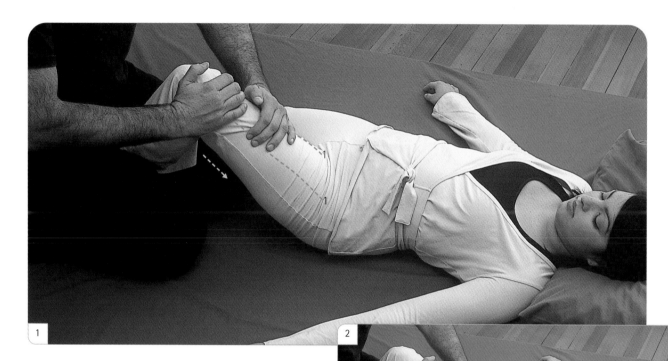

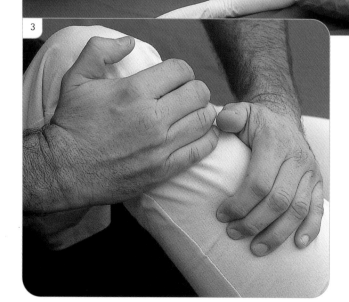

If your client is a woman, work on her left leg first. Kneel with her foot secured between your knees, her knee bent and raised. Place both your hands on the thigh above her knee as indicated.

1 Your right palm is on energy line 1 of her outer leg and the fingertips of your right hand are on energy line 1 of her inner leg, while your left fingertips are on the first energy line of the outer leg.

2 3 With your elbows pointing out slightly, rhythmically hook and pull into the thigh muscle as you move up the thigh with alternating hands, and then down toward the knee again. This both works the energy line and loosens the muscle. The pulling force should not come from your biceps but rather from you moving your trunk a little from side to side and leaning back slightly.

PALM PRESSES ON THE THIGH

Place the client's heel as close to her buttock as possible.
1 Interlace your fingers and place them on the client's thigh so that the palm heels are positioned over energy line 2 on both the inner and outer thigh. Press and squeeze the palms toward each other, as if you were operating a very large nutcracker — but gently! 2 3 Work your way up the thigh to just before the groin and back again.

4 When your hands are once again just above the knee, lean back with your upper body. If the client's leg is correctly positioned, her body will move fairly freely, with her posterior lifting off the mat. Create a feeling of connection with your client's body as you lean back.

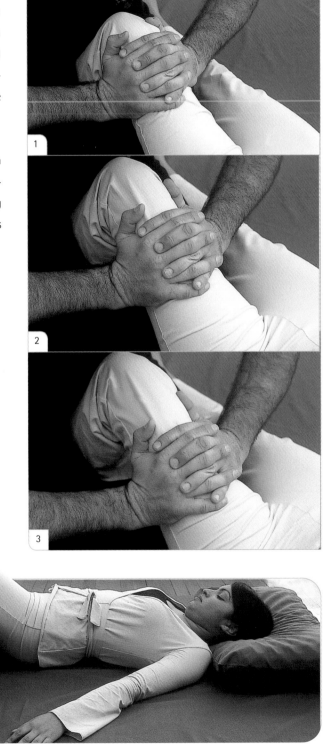

PROCEDURE ⬭ **16**

CALF WORK

With the client's foot gripped between your knees and you facing her shin, ☐1 wrap your hands around the back of her calf just below the knee, your fingertips touching each other.

Once again, using your body weight, lean back and pull toward you. Reposition both hands 3cm (1in) or so lower on the calf muscle and repeat. Proceed like this all the way down to the Achilles tendon and up again.

Now, keeping the fingers hooked behind the calf, with alternate hands walk the fingertips first down, then up the calf, pulling toward you. Then interlace your fingers and squeeze the calf muscle, using a nutcracker-like palm press to pull the muscle away from the bone. Lean

forward so you're pulling away from you. Repeat up and down the calf muscle.

PROCEDURE 17 Now for some thigh work: your client's foot is still secured between your knees. ☐2 Interlock your fingers, leaving thumbs free. Use the pads of your thumbs to press gently on energy line 3 to either side of her leg. Hold the pressure for a few seconds on each pressure point. ☐3 Work your way up and down the thigh as before.

☐4 By varying the tightness of your interlaced fingers, you can adjust the position of your grip to make sure that the thumbs are moving precisely along the third energy line.

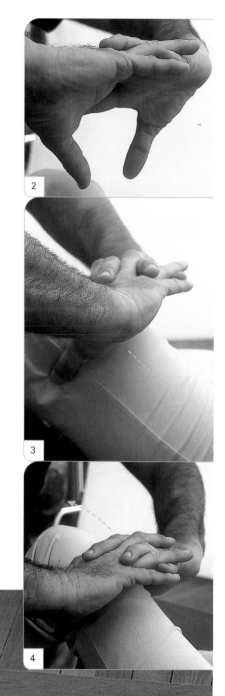

1

2

3

4

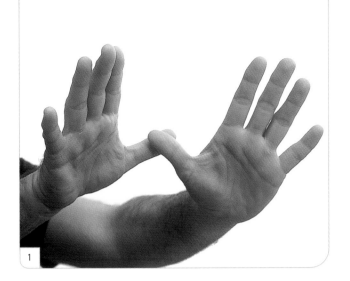

SCISSOR THUMB PRESSES

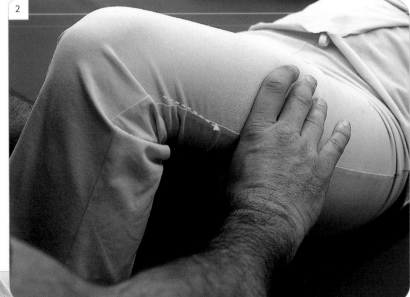

Loosen your interlocking fingers a little more so you can reach the centreline on the back of the client's thigh. 1 Place one thumb on top of the other as indicated to allow for a firmer pressure into the muscle. 2 3 Keeping your thumbs on track by sliding along the thigh with your fingertips, push into the centreline from behind the knee to the buttock and back again (the inside hand could stop mid-thigh). Do an alternating thumb walk up and down the line.

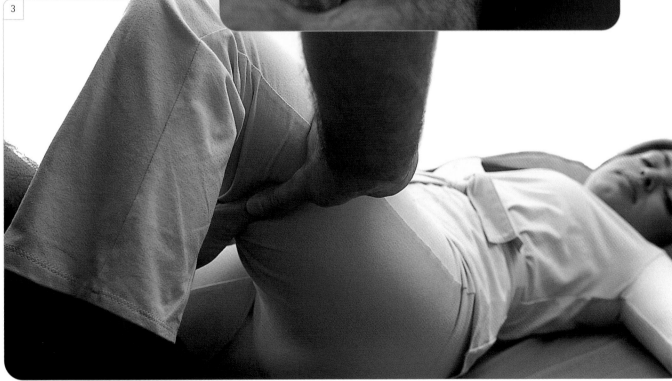

HAMSTRING STRETCH

Half-kneel on the mat with the client's foot positioned against your upper thigh as indicated in the photo (the sequence shows the final hand position of the practitioner in this particular procedure). Your hand cups and supports the knee of the client's bent leg. Your other hand presses gently down on the thigh of her extended leg, just below the groin area.

Slowly rock your body forward, pushing her knee as close to her chest as it will comfortably go. Hold the stretch for a few seconds. Rock back into your starting position and move your palm down to the middle of her thigh. Rock forward again and attempt to increase the stretch a little. Hold for a few seconds, then rock back to the beginning position.

1 Now press down with the palm just above the knee. 2 Rock forward again into the stretch. Work your way back through the procedure by repeating the stretch with the hand at mid-thigh and then just below the groin.

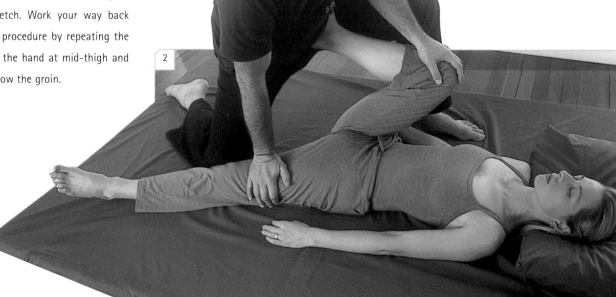

HIP STRETCH

Open your kneeling stance outward to allow you to open out the client's bent leg as well. To prevent her body from moving too much, you can pin the straight leg in position by hooking your foot over her ankle. To begin, cup your client's knee with one hand. Use the other to palm press along the inner thigh from the knee to just short of the groin and back again.

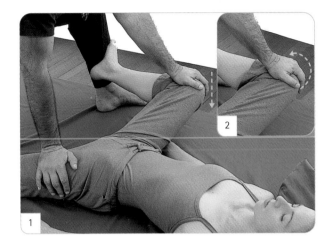

1 Next, place that palm on the hip area of the client's extended leg and gently press down on the opposite cupped knee, thereby executing a very effective groin stretch. Do this very slowly and gently, and keep on asking the client for feedback.

2 Then rock the client's bent leg from side to side, as if you were drawing a semi-circle in the air with her kneecap. This promotes energy flow in the client's hip joint and can increase the range of motion around the hip.

3 Fold her leg across her body, holding her torso in place with one hand placed gently on her floating ribs. With the other hand, push down on the leg to execute a very strong stretch to the buttock muscles (gluteus). Be extremely careful when doing all the leg stretches and continually ask the client for feedback.

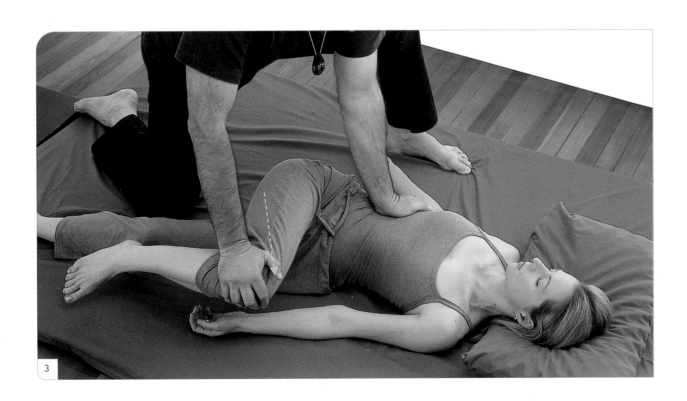

LEG STRETCHES

Raise the client's leg vertically and cup her heel or hold her leg around the ankle with one hand. Position your other hand behind her knee. [1] For the first stretch, simply try to press the knee of the almost fully extended leg to her chest.

Then try to straighten the client's leg diagonally toward the opposite shoulder. [2] Once again, to prevent the client's body from raising up off the mat, hook the instep of your back foot over her shin (this is an option; it may be too strong a stretch for the client or uncomfortable for the practitioner). Do a sequence of five of these stretches, moving the hand from the back of the knee to mid-thigh, to the upper thigh, then back to mid-thigh and the back of the knee once more.

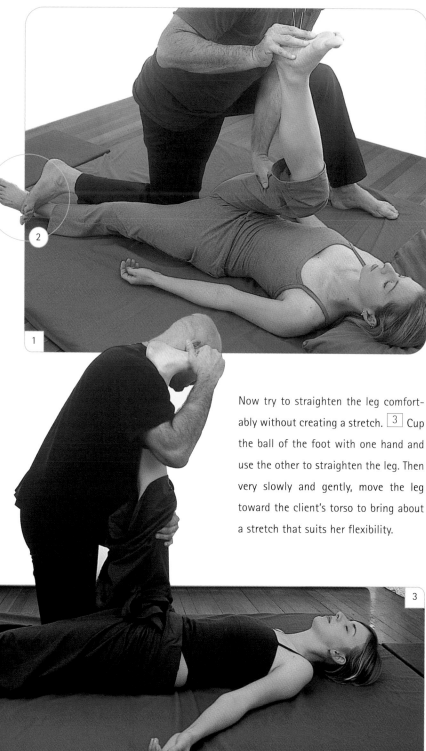

Now try to straighten the leg comfortably without creating a stretch. [3] Cup the ball of the foot with one hand and use the other to straighten the leg. Then very slowly and gently, move the leg toward the client's torso to bring about a stretch that suits her flexibility.

THIGH RELEASE

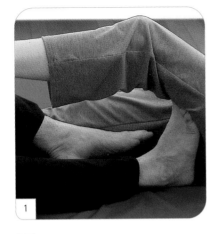

1 Sit back, lowering the client's leg but keeping it bent at the knee so that you can place the ball of your one foot against the back of her thigh, just below the knee. Hold her foot securely with your hands, one hand cupping the heel, the other holding the instep with the fingers resting on top of the foot. Extend your leg, pushing into the client's thigh with the sole of your foot. 2 Lean back and hold for 10 seconds. You can create a great deal of leverage and effect a deep release in the muscles of the back of the thigh and buttock (gluteus).

3 Now form a 90-degree angle between her thigh and calf and push her knee toward her chest. This causes her upper thigh to ride up slightly and the ball of your foot naturally moves to her buttock, or very close to it. Lean back and hold for 10 seconds. Move forward and again push her knee toward her chest. The ball of your foot naturally repositions on her sitting bone, so lean backward once more. As your foot changes position, you release the muscles from her mid-thigh all the way to the buttock.

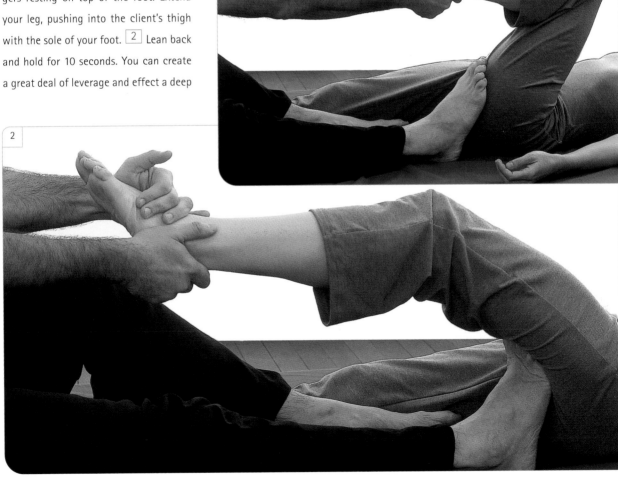

ANGLED LEG STRETCH

1 To transition smoothly from the previous technique, the client's foot is placed angled out to the side of her buttock. The other leg is extended. Press the knee down as far as it will comfortably go. Note that many clients will not have the flexibility for the bent knee to touch the ground. This is not a problem — simply use a firm cushion to support the leg, and in the case of the chopping technique, sit so that you are supporting her leg on your thigh. Do the same sequence of palm presses and butterfly palm presses as you did in procedure 11, p45.

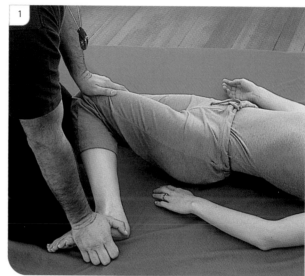

2 Once you have done this, gently press your palms together. Fan out the fingers, leaving space between each pair. 3 4 Keeping wrists loose and relaxed, chop down the thigh and calf and up again. Repeat this two or three times. Carefully lift up the client's bent leg, straighten it and gently do some palm circles around the knee.

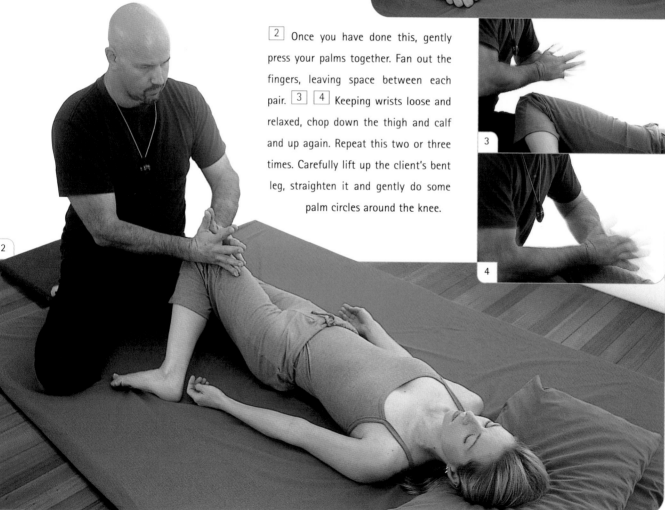

BACK-OF-LEG STRETCH

1 Position yourself on the outside of the client's leg in a half-kneeling posture as indicated (depending on your own comfort level, you could half-kneel with either leg). Rest your client's leg on your kneeling thigh. Your hand cups her foot, fingers on her Achilles tendon. The ball of her foot and her toes push against your forearm. Use your other hand to palm press up and down the upper thigh, simultaneously using a rocking motion to create a stretch by pressing the foot toward her body. Ninety per cent of this technique's effect lies in the stretch, while the palm pressure accounts for only 10 per cent.

Change to the client's other leg and go through procedures 11 to 24 on that leg.

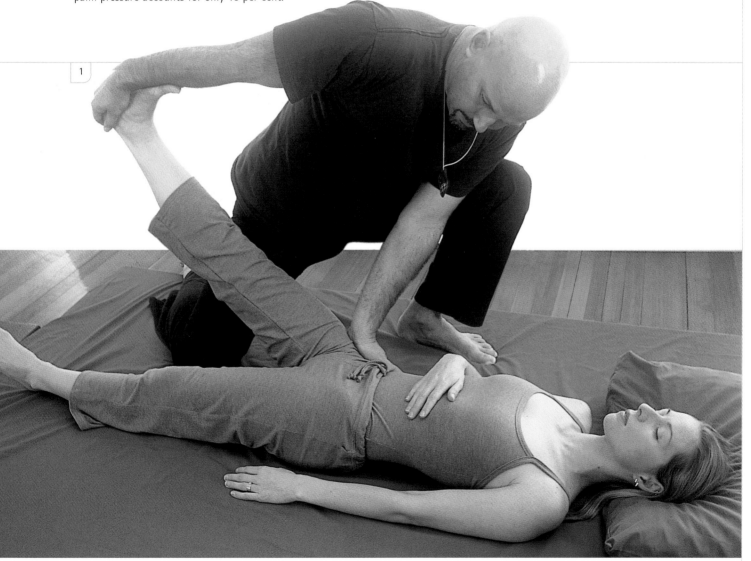

SHOULDER STAND

has been used for this particular client's comfort; generally, do not use one.) Rocking forward in your stance, use the lever of his legs to easily move him into a type of shoulder stand. Although it looks difficult and strenuous, if done correctly very little effort is required on the part of the practitioner or client.

3 Ask the client to relax his elbows and the hands on his knees. Rock forward again, placing him into a position similar to the Plough pose of yoga. Stand fairly close to the client for this, as too much distance between yourself and the client could cause you to hurt your back!

This technique was clearly adapted from Hatha Yoga. (In both yoga and Thai massage, it's believed that inversion of the body for short lengths of time has a very positive effect on blood circulation and energy flow.)

1 Raise your client's legs. Support them so that they form a 90-degree angle to the client's torso. (This prepares him or her for the next two slightly more strenuous steps.)

2 Ask the client to put his hands on his knees, keeping the arms extended and locked at the elbows. This makes of the body a single, very stable structure. (Note: the cushion

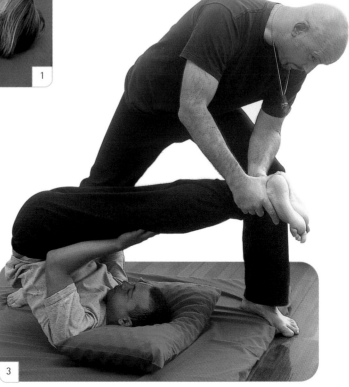

LOOSENING HAMSTRINGS & HIPS

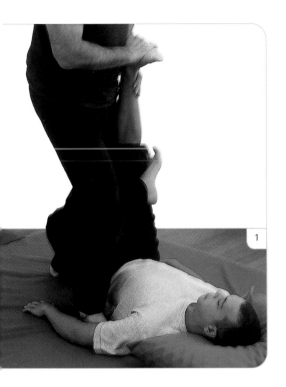

times to warm up the area, then use the tip of your elbow to press downward into the pressure points (see p36). Maintain the pressure for five seconds on each point. Do all six points two or three times. In-between moving from point to point, straighten your arm after applying pressure for five seconds. This prevents you from tensing up and smoothly reduces the pressure on the client's sole. Be gentle: you can apply a lot of force in this position.

Then unlock your foot position and step back. Your one hand cups his foot at the heel or supports his ankle, keeping his leg extended, while your other hand makes a very loose fist. 2 3 Keeping both hand and wrist relaxed, gently strike the entire back of the thigh and calf. This is very relaxing, especially after the 'pain' of the pressure points.

Separate your client's legs, bending the knee of one so that the ankle rests on the thigh, just above the knee, of the extended leg. 1 Step over his bent leg, gently 'locking in' both his legs. Now rock forward and backward in your stance three times, increasing the extension of your rocking motion each time.

If the client is flexible, simply move your back leg in, placing it up against his buttock. If he is not flexible or you are too tall, shift yourself around the client's extended leg so that you have access to the pressure points on the sole of his extended foot. Your one hand supports the client's leg at the ankle. You can roll the forearm across the bottom of the upturned sole of his foot two or three

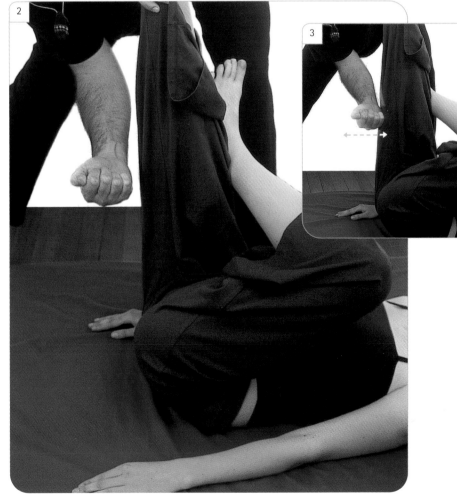

PROCEDURE 27

PRESSURE POINTS ON FOOT

1 Your client lies with one leg at right angles to her extended leg, ankle resting on the knee. If the client is flexible, move your back leg up from its supportive position in the previous technique and step over the client's bent leg, placing it up against her buttock. If this is awkward for you, shift yourself around the client's vertically extended leg so that you have access to the pressure points on the sole of the foot.

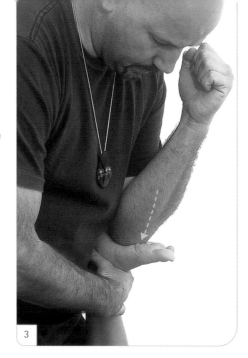

2 Your one hand holds and supports the client's leg at the top of the ankle. You can roll your forearm across the bottom of the client's foot two or three times to warm up the area, then use the tip of your elbow to press downward into the six pressure points of the foot. 3 Maintain the pressure for five seconds on each point. Do all six points two or three times. Straighten your arm each time you hold the pressure for five seconds. This prevents you from tensing up and reduces the pressure on the foot. Be gentle; you can generate a lot of force in this position. Next, step out of the pose back over her crossed leg. Hold her foot cupped at the heel with your one hand, thereby keeping her leg extended. With your other hand, make a very loose fist. Keeping both fist and wrist relaxed, gently strike the entire back of the thigh and calf.

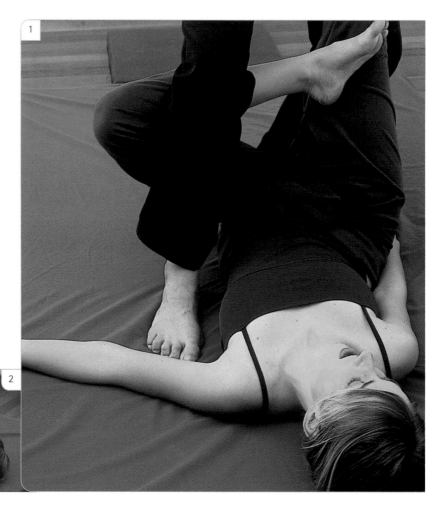

GLUTEUS MUSCLE STRETCH

Depending on your height, you may be able to do this in a slightly bent standing position or you may need to kneel as indicated. 1 Without changing the client's vertical leg posture, position yourself so that the Achilles tendon of the client's extended leg rests on your shoulder. Your one hand supports the client's bent knee, the other grasps his ankle (or sole). 2 Rock forward and backward five times. You can use your hand on his knee or pressing against the thigh of his bent leg to assist his stretch

as you rock forwar straighten both of t gently, reposition opposite sides an procedures 26 to 28 other leg.

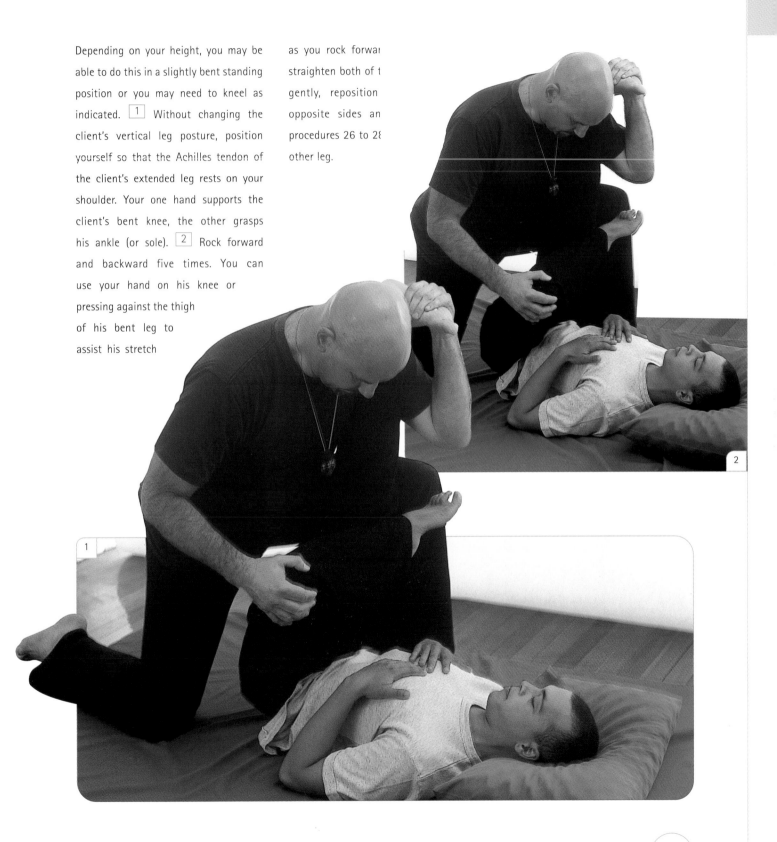

HAMSTRING RELEASE

1 Raise both of the client's legs, gently bending them so that his knees are as close to his chest as he can manage. Depending on your height, you may have to take quite a wide stance, with your knees collapsed forward. If you are tall and experience knee problems, avoid this technique. Otherwise, your feet should be positioned at the same width as your knees, which press on the gluteus muscles (buttock) at the 'sitting bones'. Both your hands support his heels.

2 Now rock forward onto the balls of your feet, creating pressure on the hamstrings. Rock back onto your feet, pulling his legs slightly toward you. Your knees are now slightly higher up the back of his thighs. Rock forward and back once more. Pull his legs closer, reposition

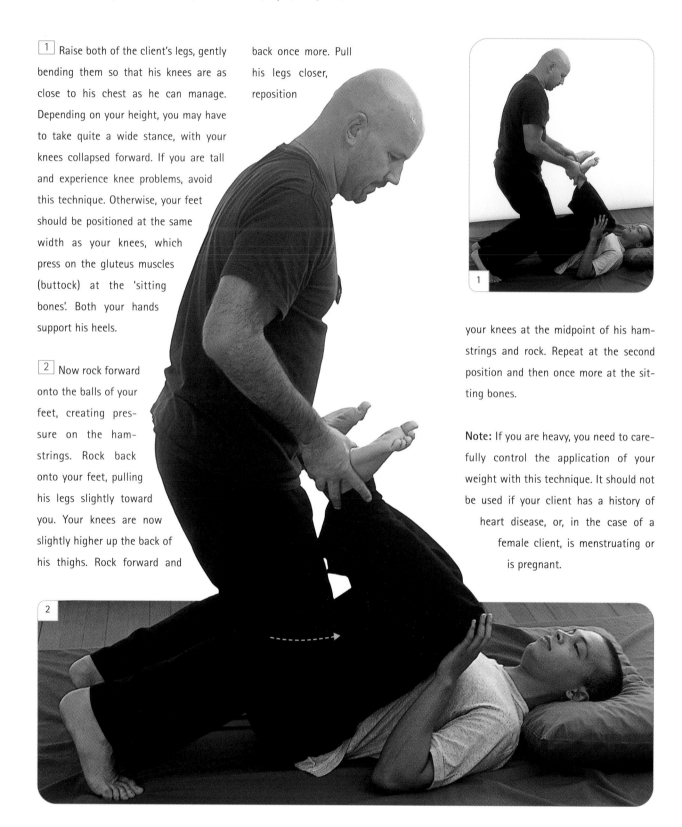

your knees at the midpoint of his hamstrings and rock. Repeat at the second position and then once more at the sitting bones.

Note: If you are heavy, you need to carefully control the application of your weight with this technique. It should not be used if your client has a history of heart disease, or, in the case of a female client, is menstruating or is pregnant.

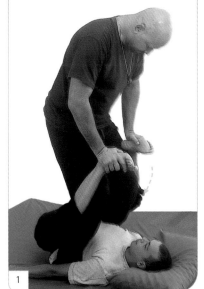

1

BACK STRETCH

2 Walk back half a step so your ankles are at the level of his hip bones. Press his legs straight down and forward.

1 Ask the client to place his arms alongside his body; his legs are raised. Holding onto the client's feet, step through his legs and place your feet next to his ribcage, your toes close to his armpits. If the client is not very flexible, hold the legs open; if the client is very flexible, press the soles of the feet together. Squat as you press the feet forward, creating a counterbalance while you rock forward three times.

PROCEDURE 31 Step back and, holding your client's feet, cross his legs by crossing your arms. Normally, the edges of his feet should rest below your knees. 3 Clasp his wrists, while he simultaneously grips yours. 4 Lean back and gently straighten your legs; your body weight will pull the client upward. Then gently lower him to the mat again.

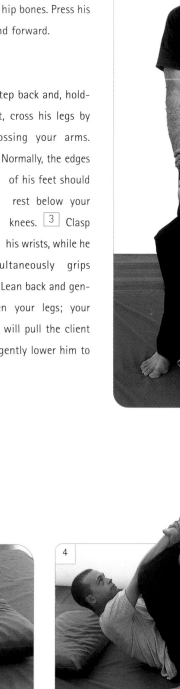

3

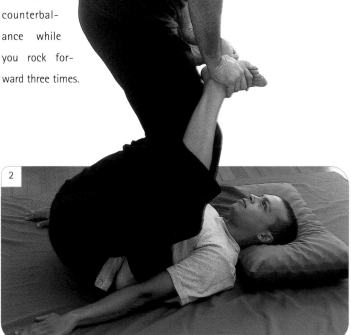

2

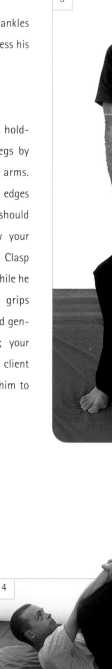

4

AB MASSAGE

Make sure you are well versed in the contraindications for abdominal massage. The client lies in a relaxed posture, legs shoulder width apart, arms outstretched, away from the body.

1 Place the fingertips of one hand onto pressure point 1 (below the navel). Place your other hand on top, supporting it. Both palms form a strong triangular wedge. Ask the client to breathe in.

2 As she exhales, press downward with the fingers and hold. Keep your hand there while the client inhales again. As the client exhales, push again, but this time

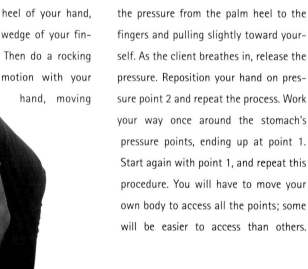

Now, once again using the navel as the centre, imagine six points on the client's belly, arranged in pairs. The top two are at a 45-degree diagonal out from the navel, the bottom two at a 45-degree diagonal below the navel. The distance from the navel to each of these four points equals the length of the client's thumb. The other two points are next to the navel, each one at a distance of half the length of the client's thumb.

downward with the heel of your hand, more than with the wedge of your fingers. Then do a rocking motion with your hand, moving

the pressure from the palm heel to the fingers and pulling slightly toward yourself. As the client breathes in, release the pressure. Reposition your hand on pressure point 2 and repeat the process. Work your way once around the stomach's pressure points, ending up at point 1. Start again with point 1, and repeat this procedure. You will have to move your own body to access all the points; some will be easier to access than others.

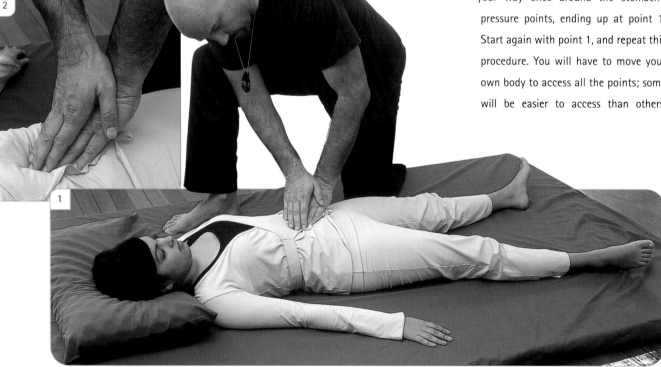

AB THUMB PRESSES

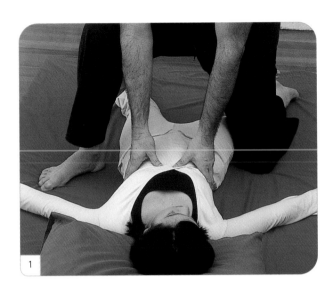

After the intensity of working the points and the scooping, relax the client with gentle palm circles on the belly area. If you wish to promote the digestive process, work the points in a clockwise direction.

1 Sitting next to the client, or half-kneeling over her, work these points with thumb presses.

2 Your fingers are on the client's sides, just below the ribs.

3 Using one thumb on each point, simultaneously thumb press points 1 and 2. Hold the pressure for five seconds or for the duration of one breath. Now thumb press points 3 and 4 — to either side of the navel — for five seconds, then points 5 and 6. Work back to 3 and 4, then 1 and 2. Move once more down to 3 and 4, finishing with 5 and 6.

Constantly ask the client for feedback and adjust your pressure accordingly. After working the nine points, you can 'knead' and 'scoop' the flesh of the belly area, with your palm into the centre, in a clockwise direction.

4 To conclude the abdominal massage, do a series of gentle palm circles.

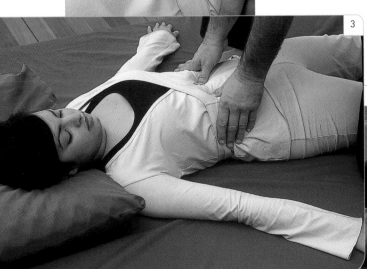

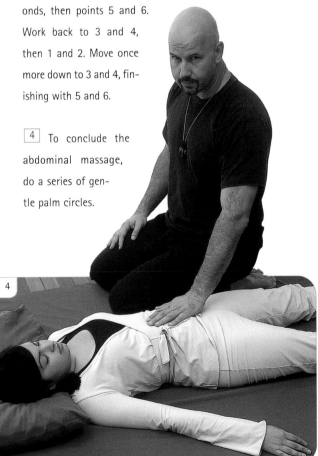

ENERGY LINES OF INNER ARMS

The client lies on her back, arms alongside her body. You may opt to move the client's arm a little further from the body to allow easier access to it. With one hand on the armpit and the other on the client's hand, stretch the arm out. 1 From this hand positioning, walk both palms inward. When they get to the elbow walk them outward again. Move them inward once more, 2 then move both hands toward the client's hand, making sure not to exert pressure on the elbow joint.

3 Now do walking thumb presses up the middle of the forearm. Avoid the elbow. Continue with the thumb presses, working between the bicep and the bone. You are working the inside energy line of the arm.

4 Then do thumb presses down the same energy line you worked up.

To continue this process, use alternating palm presses all the way up the arm and all the way down again.

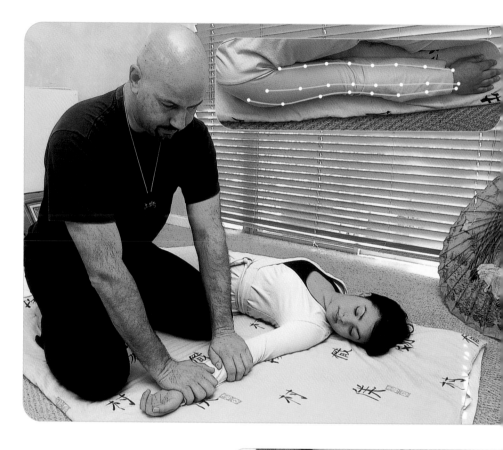

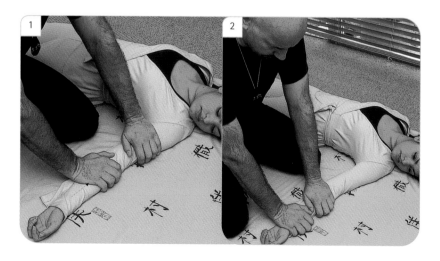

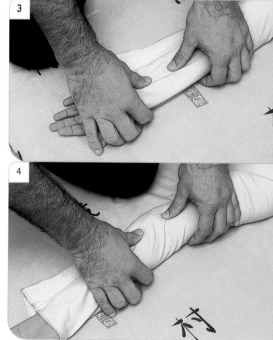

ENERGY LINES ON OUTER ARMS

Place the arm to be worked on close to the client's body. Put your one hand on her shoulder, the other one on her wrist, and stretch the arm out. As you did on the inside of the arm, work with palm presses moving inward to the elbow, then move away and back to the elbow again, finishing with both palms working down to the hand.

1 2 Do walking thumb presses up the centre of the forearm, avoiding the elbow, then continue up the centre of the outer upper arm. 3 4 Return the same way with your thumb presses. Finish with alternating palm presses up the arm, then down again.

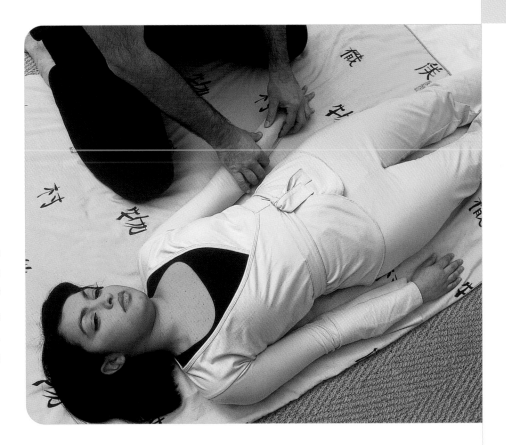

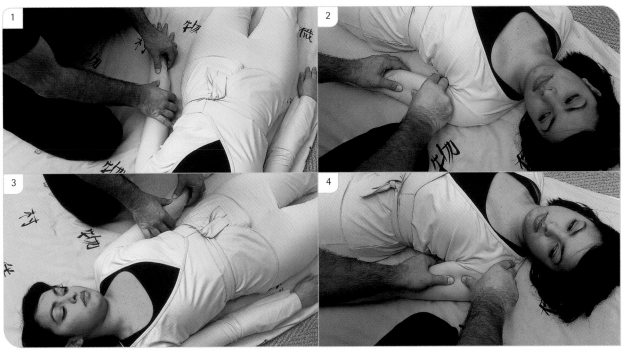

PALM WORK

This side-lying position can be used as an alternative to the supine pose. To warm up the client's hand, pick it up with both of yours and hold it so that her palm is facing the floor. Your thumbs are next to each other, on the top of her wrist. Knead the palms of her hands by moving your little fingers closer to each other and apart again. Move your hands up and down hers as you knead.

1 2 Now, interlace your fingers with hers as illustrated. This allows you secure but comfortable control of her palm. You have several options for working her palms with your thumbs. You can use a six- or eight-point pattern similar to that of the abdominal massage. 3 Both thumbs can access pairs of points at the same time or 4 you can alternate. You can also do the Michael Jackson 'moonwalk' in which you alternate pulling the thumbs across her palm toward you. In-between any of the techniques, it's advisable to knead and rub the client's hand in a 'free form' style to relax it.

When you massaged the foot, you worked five lines on the bottom of the foot and four lines on the instep. The Thais apply the same concept to the hands. Work the five energy lines (as indicated on inset photo, above) of the palm, starting at the centre of the palm heel and working up each finger, using thumb presses. On the fingers themselves, use gentler finger circles instead of direct presses. When you get to the tip of each finger, give it a pull. Finish by kneading the whole hand again.

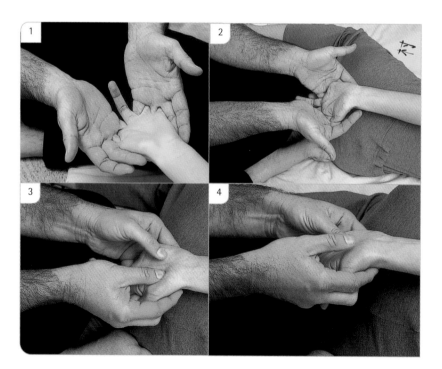

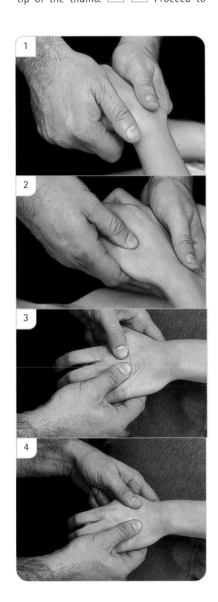

WORKING THE HANDS

work the whole back of the hand in the same manner. Finish by kneading.

5 Next, interlace your fingers with hers. Support her wrist with the other hand. 6 7 8 9 Rotate the whole hand five times in one direction and five times in the other.

Keeping your fingers interlaced, and making sure that there is no angle to her wrist when you do this, pull at the wrist. Repeat this three times, then finish off by kneading the hand.

Turn the hand over so that the palm is facing downward. Start by thumb pressing at the wrist, then do thumb circles down to the client's thumb web 1 2 and down the thumb. Press and pinch the tip of the thumb. 3 4 Proceed to

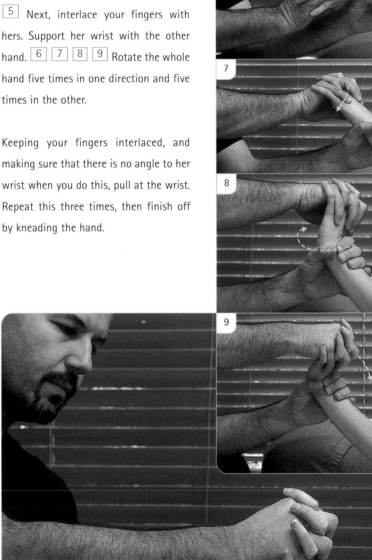

RELEASING FINGER JOINTS

The next technique 'clicks' the finger joints. Some clients may not enjoy this technique! Grab each finger individually. 1 2 You can hold her finger with your thumb and index finger or you can lock her finger between the first knuckles of your index and middle finger. This gives you a very strong grip, but may be uncomfortable for some clients. Rotate her finger one way, then the other, to loosen it up. When you feel that the finger is sufficiently relaxed, give a firm and sudden pull on it. There will usually be an audible 'click' and a pleasant feeling of release for the client.

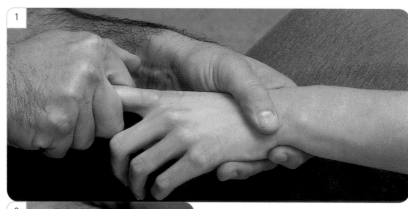

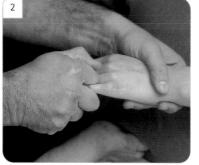

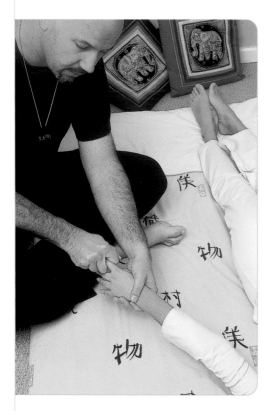

Now hold the client's hand with both of yours so that you're looking directly at her palm. With your fingers supporting the back of her hand, start with both of your thumbs at the centre of her palm.

Slide the thumbs over her palm, one going to her thumb, one to her little finger. As you slide your thumbs along the fingers, bend them as far back as you can to stretch them. Repeat the procedure on the client's index finger and the fourth finger, then on the middle finger.

To finish the work done on the hand, knead as you did previously.

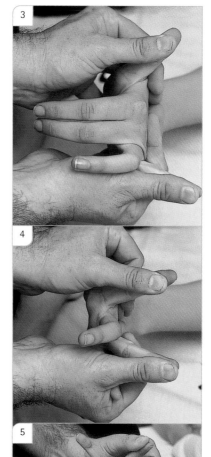

TRICEP STRETCH

1 Bend the client's arm and take it up and over to the side of his head, placing it so that the palm is flat on the floor, fingers pointing back toward his shoulder.

2 Cup his elbow with one hand, place your other hand on the top of the thigh and stretch. Move your hand to the centre of his thigh and repeat. Next, move your hand to just above the knee and stretch again. Return to the second position, then the first position, stretching each time.

Now take the hand from the thigh and place it on the client's tricep. Isolate the tricep muscle, squeeze it and lift it away from the bone with a slight twisting motion. Work your way up to the elbow and down again. Straighten your client's arm and shake it out a little.

> Now move to the other side of the client's body and repeat techniques 34 to 39.

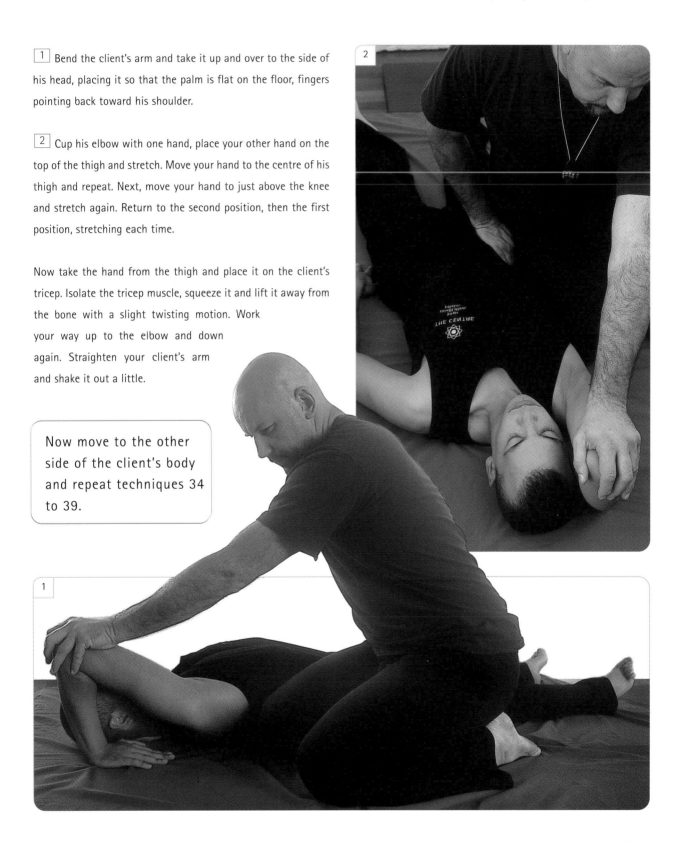

SHOULDERS, NECK AND HEAD MASSAGE

Shoulders

Sit cross-legged above your client's head. Some therapists like to rest the client's head on their lap, on a cushion. First you work the shoulders. Palm press along the top of each shoulder from the neck outward, and back in again (1-2-3-2-1). Next, apply five-second thumb presses into each trapezius muscle (triangular-shaped muscle that moves the shoulder blade), out from the neck and in again (1-2-3-2-1). Conclude with another set of five palm presses along the shoulders.

Neck

Using your fingertips, gently work the muscles of the neck, especially those responsible for holding up the neck, as they often carry a great deal of tension. It is much easier to feel specific areas of tension in the neck than in the larger and stronger muscle groups of the back. Use your fingertips to 'read' these areas of tension, and improvise to release them. Aside from finger circles, you can hook and pull with the fingers, push, and stroke. Once you start feeling the neck muscles relax, gently hold the head by curling your fingers under the occiput (the hollow at the base of the skull) and slowly pull the head slightly toward you. This creates a gentle traction and brings some relief to the cervical vertebrae.

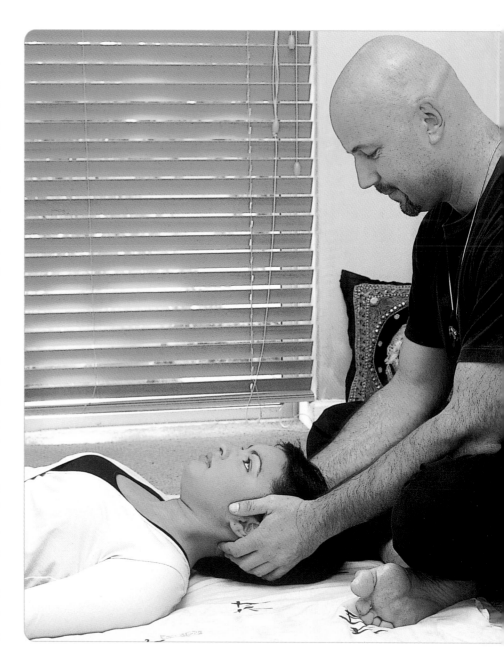

You can experiment with different techniques to find out what your client prefers. As these areas are often quite sensitive, most clients will prefer softer techniques such as finger circles rather than harder ones such as thumb presses.

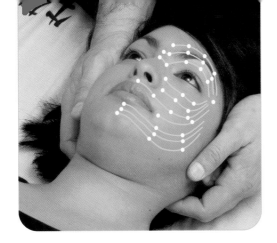

FACIAL MASSAGE

Above **The facial area showing the main pressure points and energy lines. Both sides of the face reflect the same energy pathways.**

Head

From the neck you move up to the skull. Here you use mostly finger circles and some finger and thumb presses. First, use finger circles to work the area around the occiput at the base of the skull. 1 2 Follow this with free-form finger circles over the whole skull area. You will find that certain areas such as the temples are much more sensitive than others.

3 4 After the finger circles, do alternating walking thumb presses up the centreline of the skull, starting at the forehead and going as far back as you can. When you have nearly reached the point at which the head touches the floor, reverse direction and thumb walk to the forehead again.

Next, put your thumbs together in the middle of the client's forehead, just below the hairline, 5 and stroke outward, 'ironing out' the skin. 6 Repeat slightly lower on the forehead. You should be able to do this two or three times before you have covered the entire

forehead. Explore the client's face with your fingertips, as if you were a blind person. It would be useful to do a series of facial and head massages with the eyes closed to develop the fine

sensitivity required to do a good scalp and facial massage. You will quickly learn to 'read and release' prime tension spots such as the jaw hinge, the temples and muscles around the eyes.

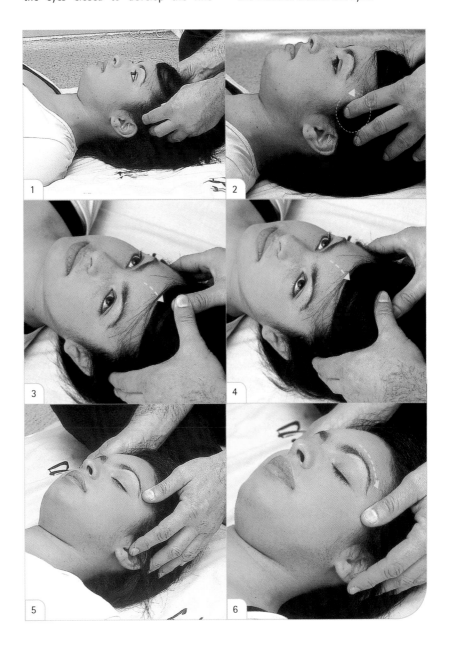

Lying on the side

SOME OF THE TECHNIQUES APPLIED TO THE LEGS while the client was lying on her back can also be done with her lying on her side. This includes holding the ankles with your hands while simultaneously applying pressure with your feet on areas of the thigh, palm presses up and down the legs, and thumb presses on the energy lines. Since these have been dealt with in the supine position; they will not be shown again here.

One very important advantage of the side-lying position is that it gives superb access to the energy lines, as these come up from the outer leg, run through the hip area, and from there run to the back. There is often a lot of stagnation in this area, which becomes evident through your client's extreme sensitivity to certain pressure points.

PROCEDURE 42

1 The client lies with the lower leg extended, her upper leg bent at right angles to it. Initially, you need to warm up the whole hip area with palm circles to create a certain degree of relaxation. Then use the fingertips of your three middle fingers to work on each of the three main pressure points. 2 3 If you cannot generate enough force, put the fingertips of one hand on top of the other. The fingertips are not necessarily flat next to each other — the middle finger is raised slightly with the outer two pushing in, creating a 'spearhead'-type formation. 4 You can now thumb press these points. Finish off by palm circling the whole area again.

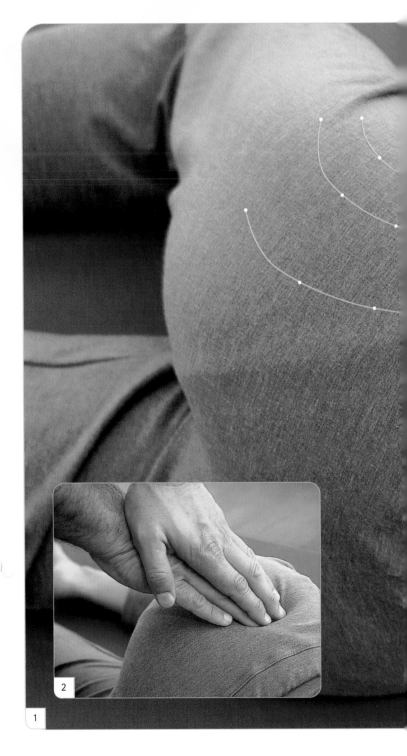

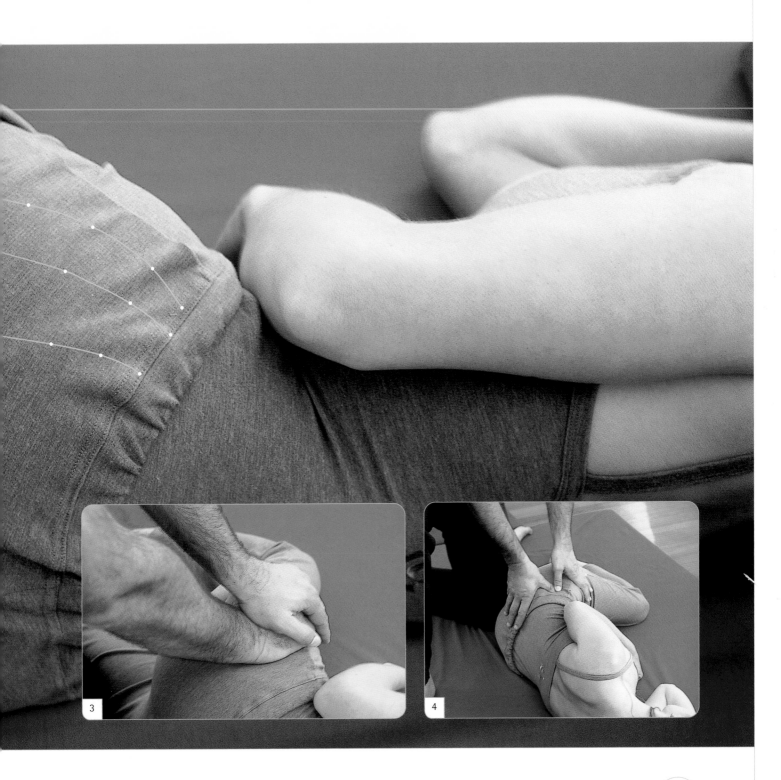

SPINAL THUMB PRESSES

Warm up the spinal erector muscles running alongside the spine by palm pressing all the way from the hip to the shoulder and back again.

1 Then do thumb presses all the way along the top edge of the spine. Your thumbs should almost touch each other as you do this. Start each thumb press by very gently feeling the spine and allowing the thumb to slide off it, then apply pressure to the muscle. (The rule about not applying pressure directly onto bone also includes the vertebrae.) Each thumb press should take about five seconds.

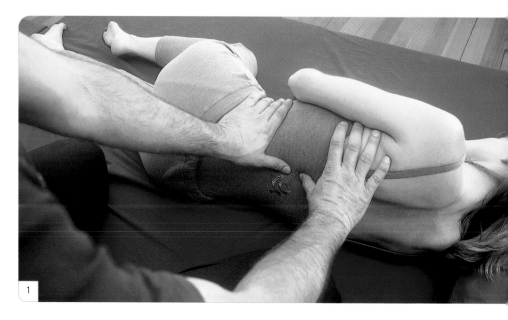

When you get to the neck, work on the scapula (shoulder blade) and the trapezius. You can ask the client to put her arm (the side that is being worked on) behind her back. 2 3 This will allow you to work your thumbs underneath her scapula quite easily. If done carefully, most clients will experience it as very pleasant. To work under the scapula, use one thumb to create pressure while your other hand stabilizes the client's shoulder.

After working the scapula, do thumb presses down the top side of the spine again. When you get to the waist, work on the points running along the waistline, i.e. at a 90-degree angle to the spine. Finish with palm presses going up and down the spine. These pressure points are still on the spinal erector muscles.

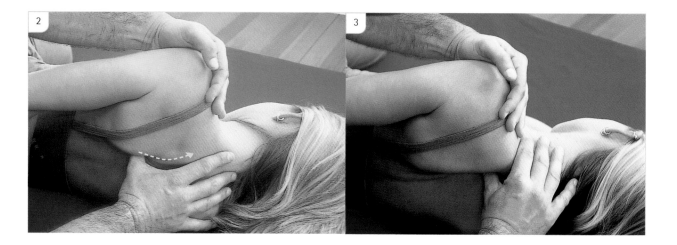

SHOULDER ROTATION

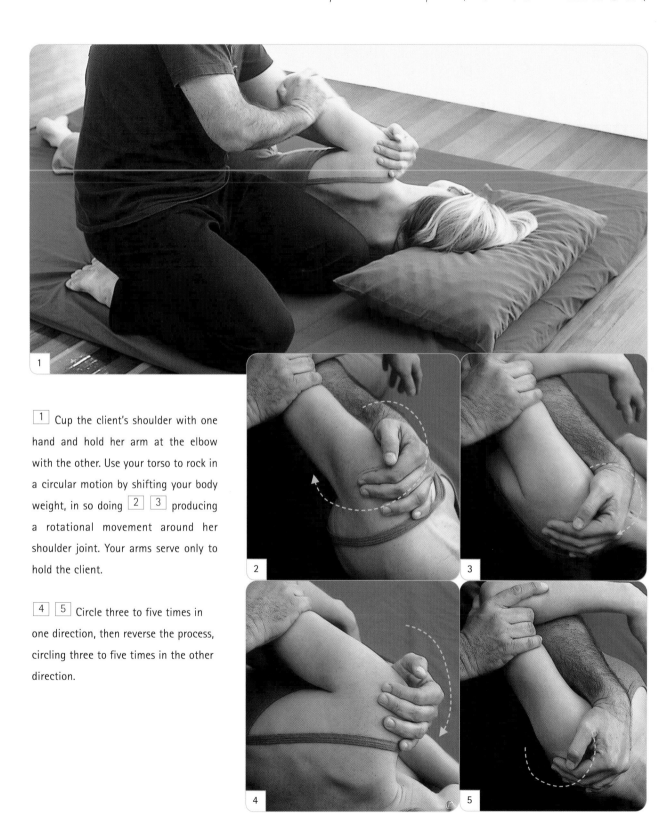

[1] Cup the client's shoulder with one hand and hold her arm at the elbow with the other. Use your torso to rock in a circular motion by shifting your body weight, in so doing [2] [3] producing a rotational movement around her shoulder joint. Your arms serve only to hold the client.

[4] [5] Circle three to five times in one direction, then reverse the process, circling three to five times in the other direction.

SHOULDER STRETCH

Position your forearm so that your elbow and upper forearm are held against the bony part of the back of your client's hip. 1 Then loop that arm under her arm and cup the front of her shoulder, or deltoid muscle.

Place your other hand over it or close to it. Use your forearm and elbow to push the client's waist forward as you 2 simultaneously pull the shoulder back with the hands.

Ninety per cent of the pressure should come from the forearm, only 10 per cent from the hands. You can vary the stretch by shifting the position of the forearm a little. You will need to keep your body quite low to the floor to achieve the correct pressure.

An equally effective variation has you holding the client's shoulder with one hand and pushing her buttock or waist with your other palm. The direction of

the push has to be parallel to the floor, not into it. Afterward, relax the waist area with palm circles to finish off.

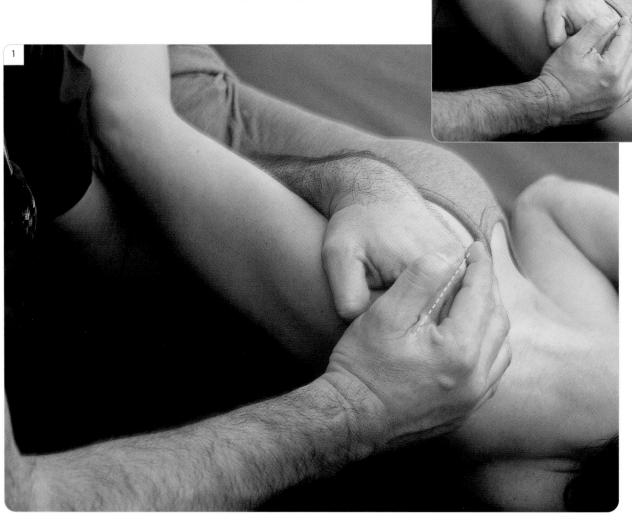

ARM STRETCH

Half-kneel behind the client. 1 Use one hand to hold her arm at her wrist; the other hand is on her armpit. Your one thigh supports her back, the other leg can support the extended arm, if required. Rock forward and stretch out the arm straight over her head. Ensure that the direction of the pull is parallel to the floor. Hold the stretch for five seconds. Rock back. 2 Reposition your hand from her armpit to the side of the client's chest. 3 4 Now move the arm in a semi-circle toward her back first, before stretching it out straight above her head. By stretching it diagonally to the rear, you can effect a strong stretch of the upper pectoral muscles.

Re-place your hand at the armpit. Now move the arm through another semicircle, this time toward the front of the client's body before stretching it out straight. Finally, relax the arm by shaking it out.

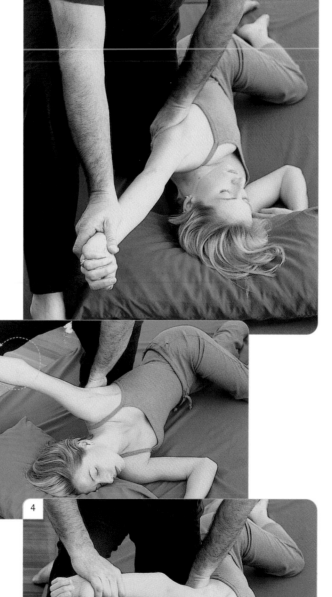

ENERGY LINES OF THE ARMS

[1] [2] [3] The energy lines of the arms can be worked in this side-lying position as an alternative to the supine position. These techniques are a repetition of techniques 34 to 39 featured on pp66–71.

LUMBAR TWIST

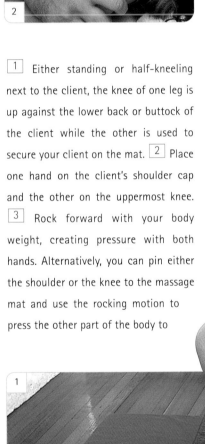

the mat. You may hear a cracking noise, indicating an adjustment in the lower back. If this is the case, do not proceed with the rest of this technique.

If there is no crack, reposition your hand mid-thigh and repeat the stretch. For the third and last stretch, reposition your leg behind the client. Keeping the one hand on her shoulder, use your palm to push forward on the client's buttock. You can brace your pushing arm against your knee and use your body to generate the force for the push.

1 Either standing or half-kneeling next to the client, the knee of one leg is up against the lower back or buttock of the client while the other is used to secure your client on the mat. 2 Place one hand on the client's shoulder cap and the other on the uppermost knee. 3 Rock forward with your body weight, creating pressure with both hands. Alternatively, you can pin either the shoulder or the knee to the massage mat and use the rocking motion to press the other part of the body to

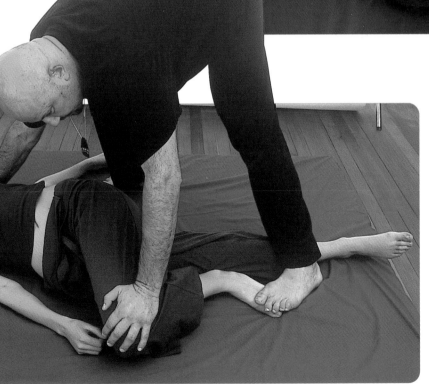

BACK AND QUADRICEP STRETCH

It is very important that you position the client correctly for the next technique to avoid injury. The client should not be lying fully on the side, but rather with the chest close to the floor so that the upward pulling motion works at the correct angle. Remember this is a stretching technique; the intention is not to apply weight to pressure points. If you are at all uncertain about your balance or your ability to correctly execute the technique, leave it out.

You can do this technique half-kneeling or standing, whichever works best for the size of your body and that of the client. ☐1 Hold the ankle of the client's lower leg with one hand and the wrist of her uppermost arm with your other. Put your foot on the client's waist to the side of her

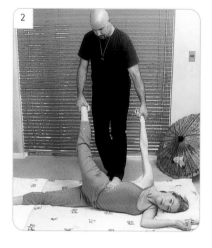

spine and pull the leg up and back. Do not pull on the arm. Don't put any weight into the foot that is on her body.

☐2 Move your foot to just below her floating ribs and pull once again. Then put the foot back into the first position and pull. Re-place your client's leg. Pick up her other leg and repeat the entire procedure.

PROCEDURE 50 Half-kneel behind the client's back. ☐3 Raise her upper leg and hold it by cupping the knee; the weight of the lower half is supported by your forearm. Cup her shoulder with your other hand, resting her arm on your thigh. ☐4 Keeping her torso steady by means of your knee placed against her lower back, create a stretch by pulling back on the leg.

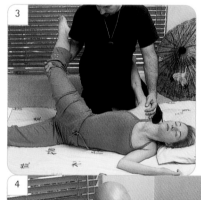

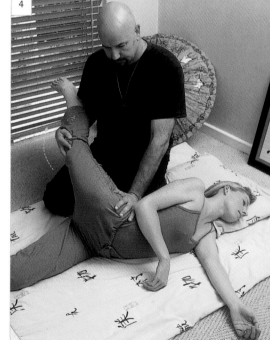

LOWER BACK STRETCH

Stand over the client with one foot next to and supporting her waist, the other behind her bent knee. The client puts her lower arm through as if she were hugging herself. 1 2 Grasp the wrist of her lower arm and ask her to grasp your wrist in turn. Bend your knees. Making sure that your back stays absolutely straight, lean back and straighten your legs, lifting your client off the floor. This technique very effectively combines gravity and a twisting stretch to effect a release and adjustments in the lower back. Relax the lower back with palm circles.

You need to be careful — keep your back straight or you may injure it. Before you do this stretch, ask the client to immediately say if she is feeling any pain; you might need to skip it.

> Now repeat techniques 42 to 51 to the other side. You could then repeat the Shoulder Stand procedure (see p58) and procedures 30 and 31. You could then either end the massage or continue to technique 52, p86.

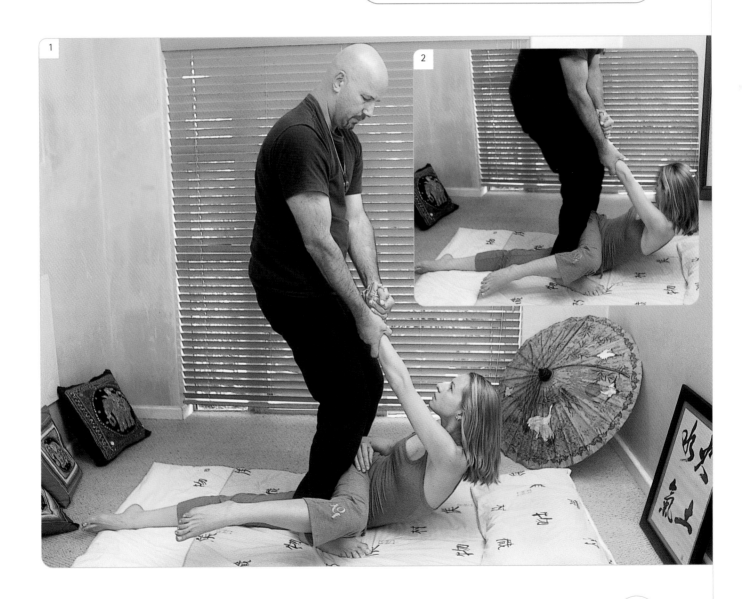

Lying on the stomach

BACK PROBLEMS ARE A COMMON COMPLAINT among a great many people. The position that allows the deepest access to the back is when the client is lying on the stomach, although it's possible to work on this area in both the seated and side-lying positions.

In Thailand, the client usually lies with the head turned to one side and his or her arms at the side. Should your client prefer this position, ask her to switch sides occasionally. It is also possible to support the forehead with a small pillow and have the face turned toward the floor. It may also be desirable to place a cushion under the abdominal area and possibly a small cushion under each instep.

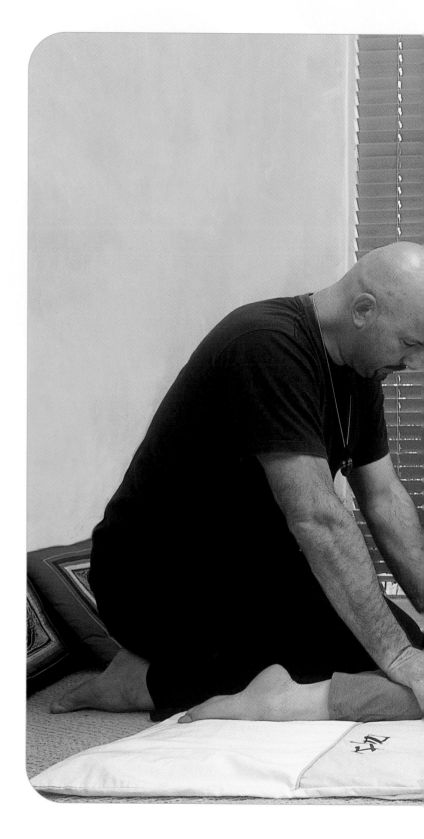

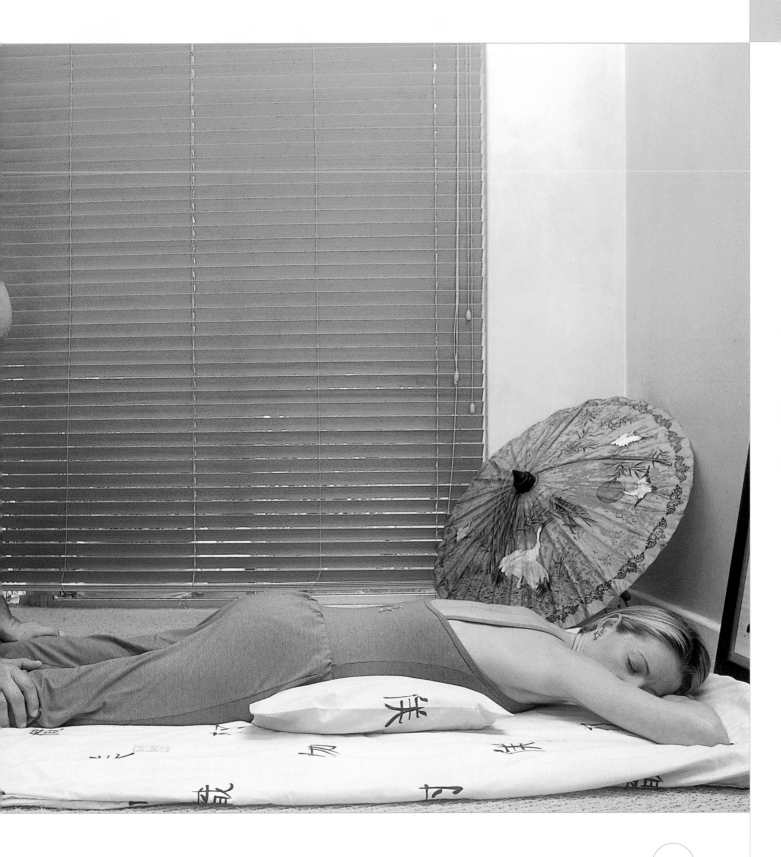

WORKING THE BACK OF THE LEGS

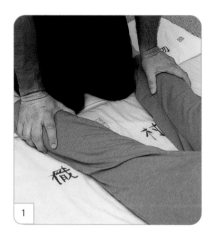

1

[1]–[3] To initiate the massage session on the legs in this position, do alternating palm presses up and then back down the entire leg — working both legs at the same time. When you reach the the back of the knees, use palm circles instead of palm presses.

[4]–[6] Having done this, stand up with your back to the client. Step back until your heels are over the soles of her feet; your heel should be just below hers. Although this technique may appear dangerous when applied by a heavy therapist on a far smaller client, you can safely regulate the amount of pressure you exert by keeping some of the weight in your toes and the balls of your feet. Deep pressure is therefore applied in a very controlled manner. Once you have settled onto the client's soles, start shifting your weight from foot to foot, moving your feet forward and backward a little. If you are concerned about creating too much pressure, use only one foot at a time and work on the lower part of your client's foot, not the heel.

You can then face the client and use the ball of your foot on her sole, either one foot at a time or both feet together. You can also kneel down, put your hands on the floor or on the client's calves to take some of your weight, and rest your knees on her soles, applying pressure by rocking from side to side. Finally, you can also 'walk' up and down her feet using alternating fists. To finish, work up and down her legs once again using alternating palm presses.

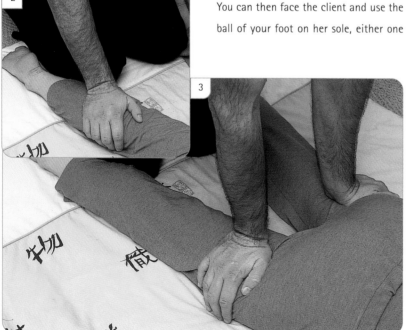

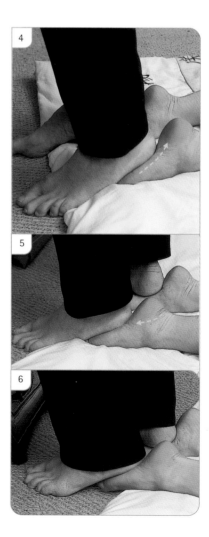

PRESSURE POINTS OF THE FEET

Half-kneel between or to the side of your client's legs. Lift her one foot and put it on your thigh, supporting the heel with your one hand. First, palm press the underside of the foot and follow up with rolling your forearm sideways over the area. 1 Then use your elbow to press the six pressure points, extending your arm to release the pressure on the client's sole after each point press. Roll your forearm over the area once more and finish off by gently striking the sole with a loosely held fist.

2 3 Kneel, rest her foot on your thigh and thumb press along the five energy lines. Use thumb circles when you get to the ball of the foot and the toes.

Next, bending the leg at the knee, push her foot toward her buttock. You can now work the lines on the instep. Start with thumb presses at the hollow of the ankle. If your client finds these too painful, use finger circles to work your way to the toes. Always use finger circles on the

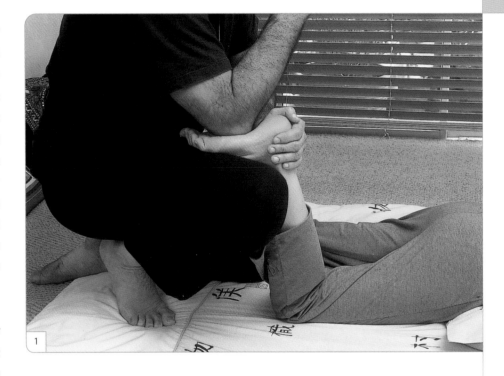

toes and conclude the work by briefly squeezing the tip of each toe.

The versatility of Thai massage becomes evident. This is essentially all the same work as that done while the client is lying on her back. You would only repeat it here if you were doing a massage of several hours' duration or if the client

needed intensive work done on the feet within the framework of a full massage. It may, however, prove to be an ideal alternative if a particular client, for one or other reason, can't be worked on in the supine position.

PROCEDURE 54   4 5 Hold her ankle with one hand, her foot with the other (see p88). Rotate the foot five times one way, five times the other. It is very important that you grip her knee between both your knees. Unlike the ankle, the knee joint is not designed for sideways movement and must not be twisted in this technique. By pinning her knee, you eliminate the possibility of this happening.

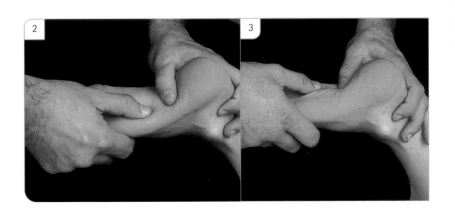

LATERAL TWIST OF ANKLE

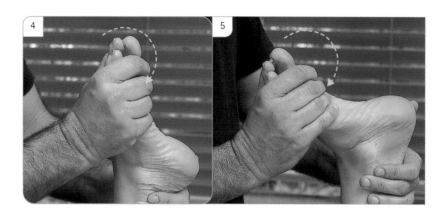

6 7 Then hold the foot as described in procedure 6, p40, supporting the ankle well, and twist (the foot, not the ankle); change hands and twist the other way.

Now repeat procedures 53–55 on the other leg.

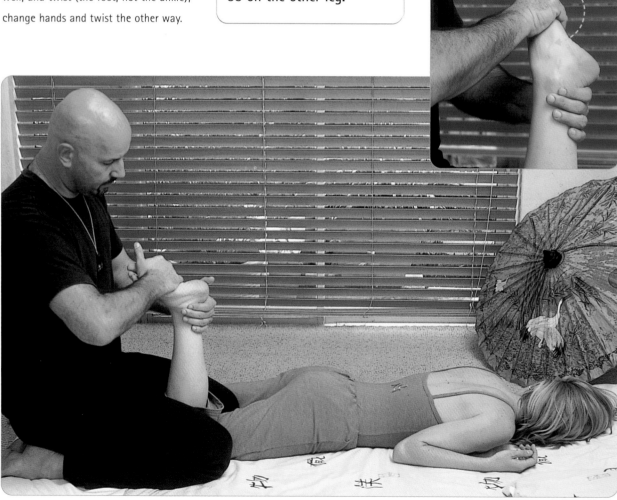

QUADRICEPS STRETCH

1 Hold both of your client's feet over the instep and bend her legs back. 2 Push her heels toward her buttocks. Do this five times, but at the first stretch hold at the ankles, then move your hand to the mid-foot, then to the toes, back to the mid-foot, and ankle again.

As a counterstretch, lift her lower leg and rest the sole of her foot along the underside of your forearm with you cupping her heel. Press downward on the foot so the heel lifts, to stretch the Achilles.

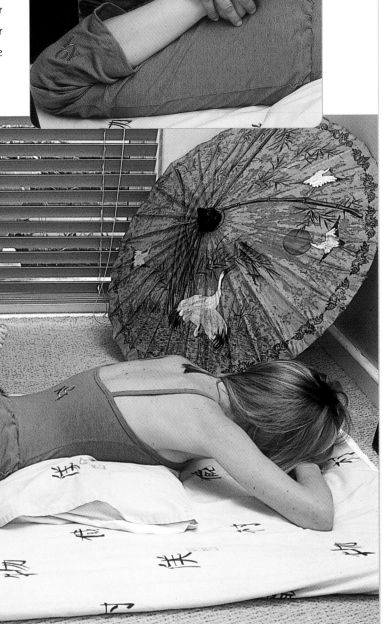

LEG STRETCH AND PALM PRESS

Open the client's legs even further and place her right foot in the crook of her left knee, or if this is uncomfortable, on the thigh above her knee. [1] With one hand hold her foot, your fingers curled over her toes, while you palm press her opposite leg, from buttock to mid-thigh to knee and back, with the other hand. At the same time, push her left foot toward her buttock. Rock forward and back to create the pressure for both the palm presses and the stretch; 70 per cent of the focus is on the leg stretch, 30 per cent on the palm presses.

QUADRICEP AND BACK STRETCH

Keeping the client's legs in exactly the same posture, reposition yourself at her side. 1 Place the knee that's closer to her shoulder on her lower back, but keep most of your weight on the ball of your foot. 2 With the hand closest to your knee, push her foot toward her buttocks, while the other hand lifts her knee. Using both hands with the gentle pressure of your knee requires a seesaw motion of your body. Move your knee up to the middle of the lower back and repeat, then to just below the ribcage, and back down the same way in a 1-2-3-2-1 sequence.

You can achieve a similar effect by using only your hands. One hand supports the client's ankle, the other one presses on the lower back as you rock.

> Repeat techniques 56 to 58, pp89–91, on the other leg as shown below.

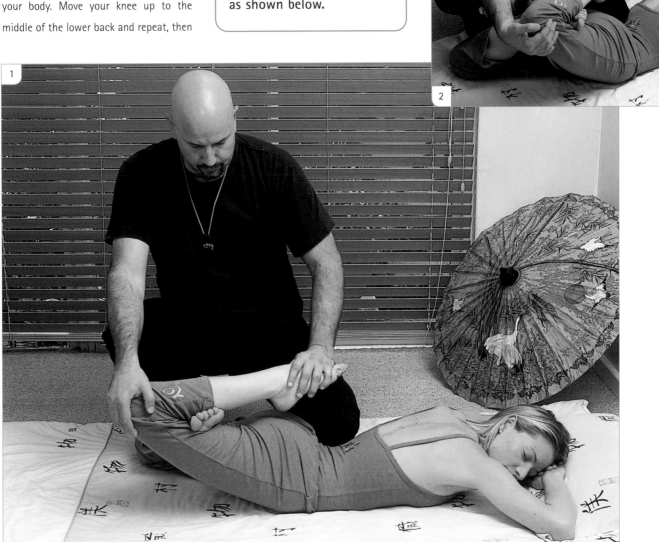

FOREARM ROLLS

Sit between the client's legs, then lift up one leg and position your thigh so that his leg rests on it. Your other leg extends straight out. Sit as close to his buttocks as possible so that you're supporting his pelvis. ☐1 Hold his ankle with one hand, resting your other forearm on his buttocks. Press your forearm down and stretch the leg by gently pulling at the ankle; hold for about five seconds. Move your forearm to the waist and stretch the leg for another five seconds.

☐2 Next, still holding the ankle, use your other forearm to roll with a side-to-side motion up the client's back to the scapula (shoulder blades), and roll back down again.

Then use both forearms simultaneously in an outward rolling motion, one forearm moving up the buttocks, the other

rolling down the calf. Move your arms first away from each other and then toward each other.

Next, bring your forearms together, one on each side of the knee, and roll them outward, working the calf and the back of the thigh. Finish off by doing the palms-together chopping technique up and down the leg.

Smoothly switch sides to work the other leg by lifting the client's leg, pivoting on your buttocks, lifting his other leg and positioning yourself underneath it.

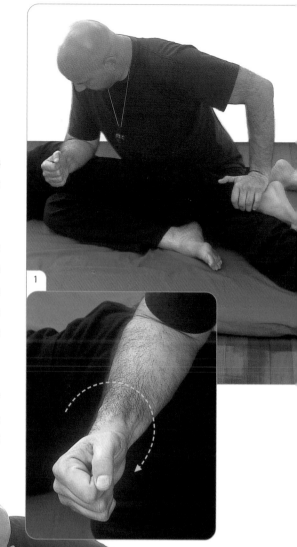

1

2

BUTTERFLY PALMS ON THE BACK

You will now work the muscles of the back in a very direct and powerful way. 1 Bend the client's legs so they form an angle at the knees and sit on the soles of his feet. This may look a little strange but is a very comfortable position for both client and therapist. Some of your weight is resting on the client's feet, some is on your own feet.

2 Palm press your way up the back, starting with butterfly palms, fingers pointing outward. As you get to the scapula, rotate the palms inward so they lie next to each other. Use a rocking motion, forward and back if you are applying pressure with both palms at the same time, side to side if you're alternating palms. You could do it one way working up the spine, the other way working down.

Take care to avoid pressure over the spine itself and limit the pressure on the scapula.

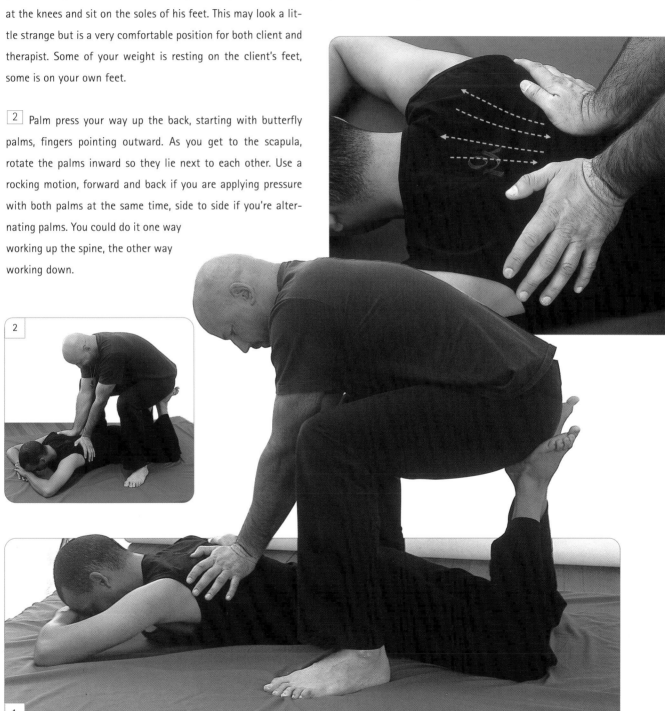

THUMB PRESSES ON THE BACK

1 Having warmed up the back with palm presses, you now do more intensive work — thumb presses up and down the back, to either side of the spine. As with the palm presses, you can work with both hands simultaneously, perhaps when you work up the back, then alternating thumbs on the way down. Use the shifting of your body weight to create the pressure required.

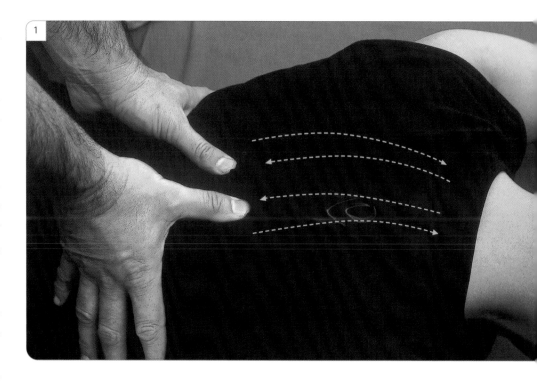

PROCEDURE 62 Do thumb presses over the client's buttocks to either side of the coccyx, then move to the points that run horizontally at the waistline (see also p76). 2 3 Work each of the three points, moving outward from the spine, asking the client for feedback. To gain deeper access to the points, ask the client to breathe in deeply, then do your thumb press to coincide with his out-breath.

PROCEDURE 63 Finally, using the ridge formed by the length of the thumb from base to tip, press your thumbs up and down the muscles running alongside the spine. Press simultaneously with both thumbs as you walk up, and alternate thumbs as you walk down.

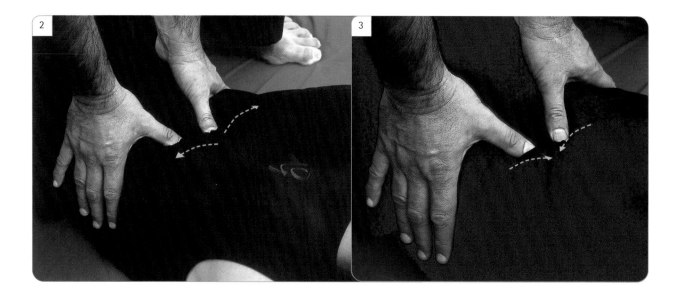

CLIENT LYING ON BACK

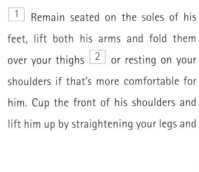

1 Remain seated on the soles of his feet, lift both his arms and fold them over your thighs 2 or resting on your shoulders if that's more comfortable for him. Cup the front of his shoulders and lift him up by straightening your legs and rocking back. Repeat three times — first softly, then stronger, and softly again. After the third stretch, gently lower the client to the mat. You can also do this while sitting on the client's buttocks.

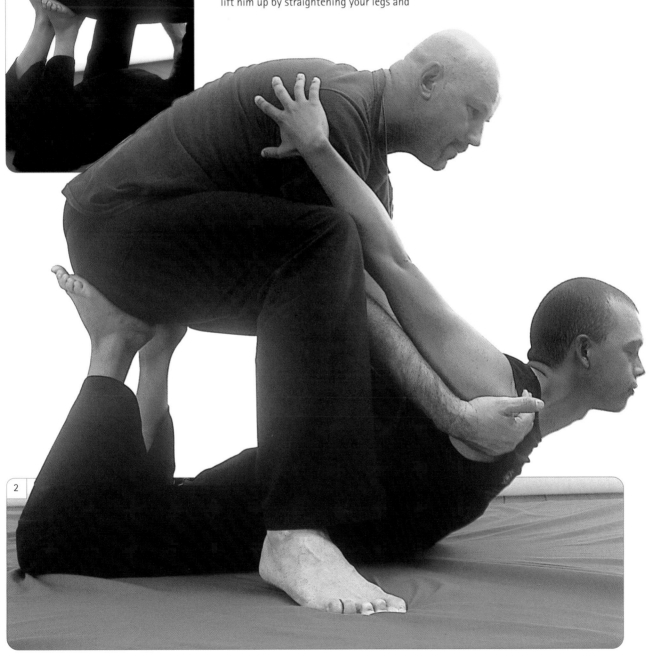

THUMB PRESSES TO SCAPULA

Half-kneel over the client; put his hand on your thigh or resting on his back if this is more comfortable. ⬜1 Using one hand to cup his shoulder, palm press the scapula and upper back with your other hand. ⬜2 Then, with the hand cupping the shoulder, pull back to create space under the edge of the scapula to do thumb presses. Do ask the client for feedback as, even though most clients find that this technique provides a feeling of deep release, it is too painful for some. Release the arm, then do palm circles around the area you've just worked. Switch your kneeling position and repeat the sequence with the client's other arm.

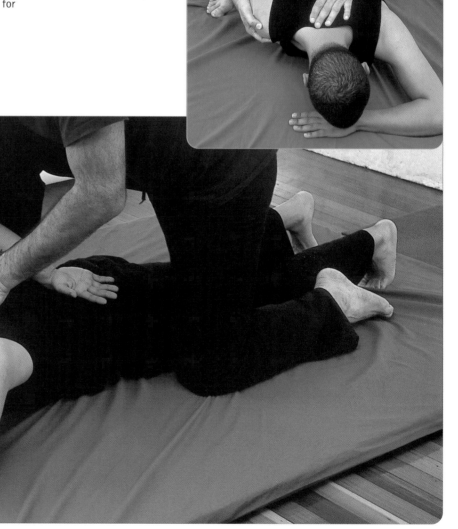

UPPER BACK STRETCH

1 Kneel against the client's buttocks, your knees positioned more or less at the sitting bones. Your feet can be inside or outside the client's legs. Your weight is mostly in your feet, not on the client. His arms lie alongside his body, palms up. 2 Pick up his arms by gripping his wrists while he grips yours. Lean back and use your body weight to pull him up. Gently lower the client.

Shift your knees so that they're positioned where leg and buttocks meet and repeat the stretch.

Then move your knees to the top of his thighs. On this last stretch you can swing the client gently to each side by pulling on one arm, then the other. Pull him back to the centre position as he looks up at the ceiling, then lower him to the mat.

To finish off, rest your knees on his buttocks again and do alternating palm presses up the arms and down the back. Continue working downward, palm pressing the backs of the legs to the ankles.

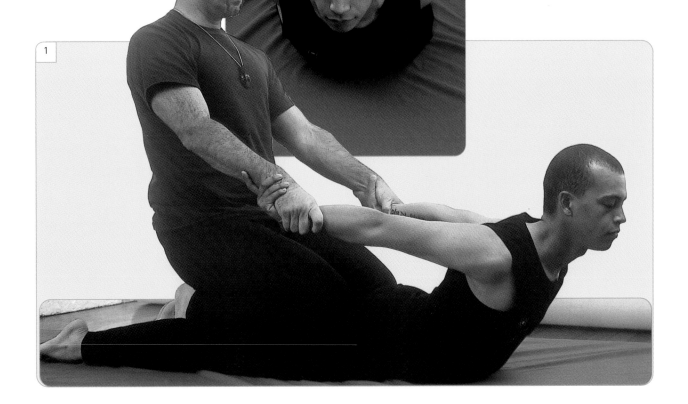

BACK STRETCH

This technique is very similar to one you have already done in the side-lying position. Maintaining a good sense of balance is important here. Stand at your client's side. Grasp his wrist with one hand (he can also grasp yours) and use your other hand to pull up the opposite leg. If your

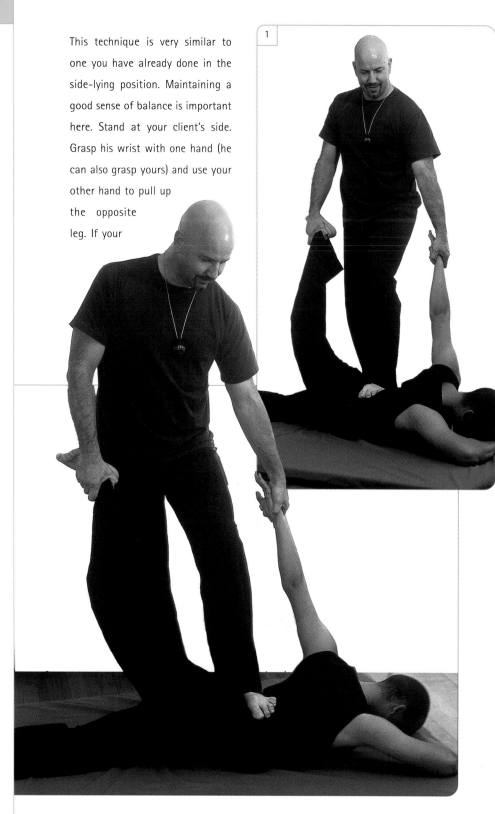

client is a woman, start with your left hand holding her left forearm, your right hand pulling on her right leg. 1 Place your foot lightly on your client's waist on the side you're working, and pull his leg up. Shift your foot up to just below his ribs and pull again. Repeat with your foot at the waist once more.

If you are finding the client's leg too heavy, you could use both hands to pull it up, as holding her arm serves only to stabilize the position. It's important that the force needed for the pull doesn't come from your arms. As you pull on the leg, slightly rotate your body around its own axis.

For the second part of the technique, pull on the leg that's closest to you. Place your foot on his waist on the same side and pull up the leg while turning your body. Repeat with your foot positioned below the ribs and again at the waist.

Now move to the other side of your client's body and repeat this sequence.

BACK RELEASE

Holding both legs at the ankles, place your one foot on the coccyx and gently pull up the legs. 1 Now place your foot on the lower back to one side of the spine and as you slightly pull up the legs, walk with your heel, applying pressure very gently, up the muscles next to the spine and down

again. Then use your other leg to repeat the technique on the other side of the spine. If you are tall, you may have to bend your supporting leg. If your client is much bigger than you are, you may find it difficult to hold up the legs.

(Note: the number and variety of techniques give you the option of leaving out any technique you feel uncomfortable with, without depriving your client.)

PROCEDURE 69 To conclude the work you've done on the back in the prone position, gently stretch out the back a little. Half-kneel next to the client. If the client is very tall, you may also do this technique standing. 2 Create a diagonal stretch along the back by placing one hand on the client's scapula and the other on the opposite buttock. Press strongly outward, moving the hands away from each other. Move your hands a little further apart and repeat, then return the hands to the original position and repeat.

Now move to the other side of the client's body and do the same stretch on that side.

Next, place one hand on the client's sacrum and the other cupped over the spine at the height of the scapula. Without exerting direct pressure on the spine, push the hands apart to stretch the back. Move the hands a little further apart, repeat the stretch then re-place hands at the first position, and repeat. Finish off with palm circles over the entire back.

At this point in the massage, you could repeat procedures 30 and 31, p63.

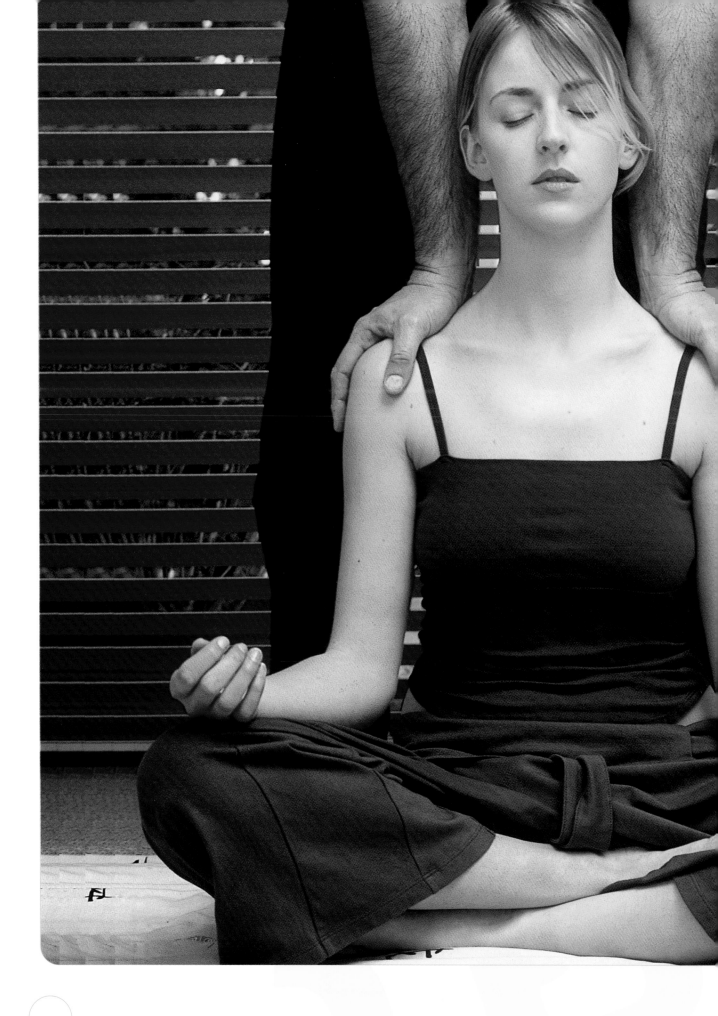

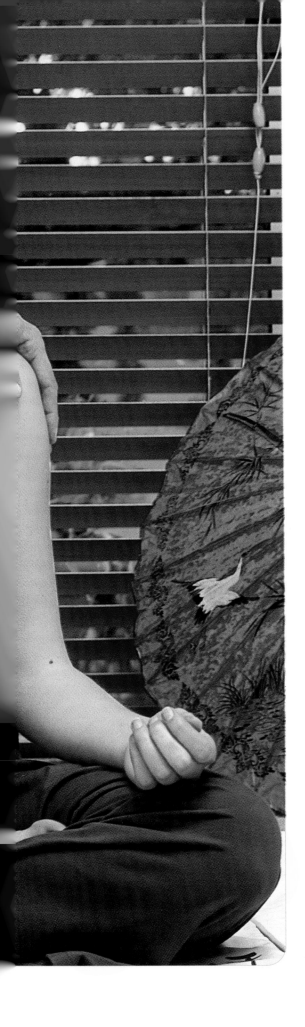

Seated upright

THE SEATED POSITION HAS VERY DEFINITE advantages and disadvantages. Its biggest advantage is that it can be done anywhere, without the use of a massage mat. It is therefore the position of choice when somebody needs an emergency massage for terrible backache after a bad day at the office or following a strenuous game of tennis. Both the seated position and the fact that Thai massage is done with both client and therapist fully dressed make this the ultimate portable massage style. No mat, table or oils are required and there is no embarrassment for the client.

A disadvantage of the seated position is that, despite you using your own body to brace or prop up the client's body, he or she needs to hold him- or herself upright. This requires muscular tension and the more tension there is, the more difficult it is to give a truly relaxing massage. Having said this, a great deal of deep and thorough work can be done on the back, shoulders, neck and head in this posture.

One thing to keep in mind is that the sequence of techniques should be seen as a guideline. Initially, while you learn, it may be useful to stick to the sequence without any deviations. As you gain experience and your sensitivity and confidence increase, you will begin to modify both the sequence and even the techniques themselves to better suit your body structure and temperament. This is a good thing. For example, when working the client's shoulders, your hands need to communicate with them. We all carry a tremendous amount of tension in our shoulder muscles. Your hands need to feel, squeeze, knead, press, push and pull until they reach some understanding of what the client's shoulders are feeling at that moment. To simply dig in, applying techniques in a textbook fashion, is not enough.

SHOULDER PALM PRESSES

1 Standing behind the client, your knee supporting her back, place your palms on her shoulders with the fingers pointing down the back. Palm press downward. Make absolutely sure the pressure is going straight down. If it is exerted at even a slight angle to the client, she will tense up the musculature of her trunk to prevent herself from being pushed over. Then palm press outward from the neck at positions 1-2-3 (see p105). Don't press directly on the bone of the outer shoulder.

2 3 Now turn your hands so that the fingers are pointing toward the front and palm press 3-2-1 inward toward the neck. It is very important that you support your client's back with your knees in this position.

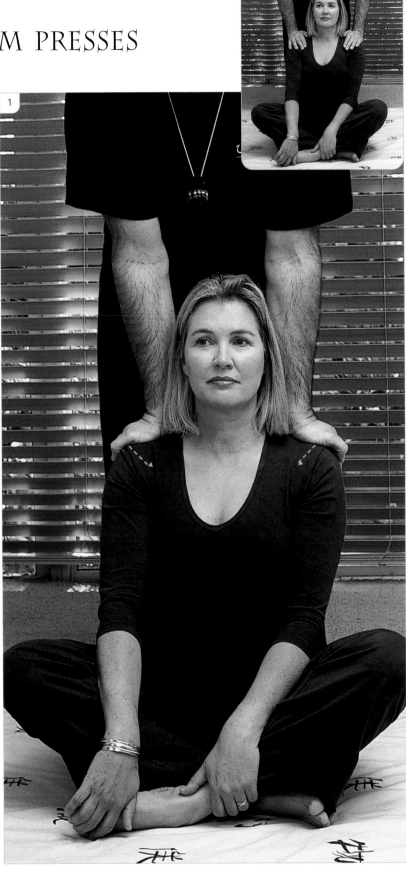

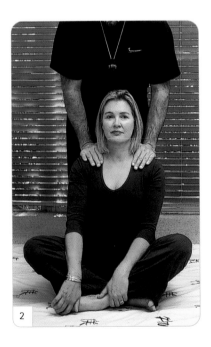

SHOULDER THUMB PRESSES

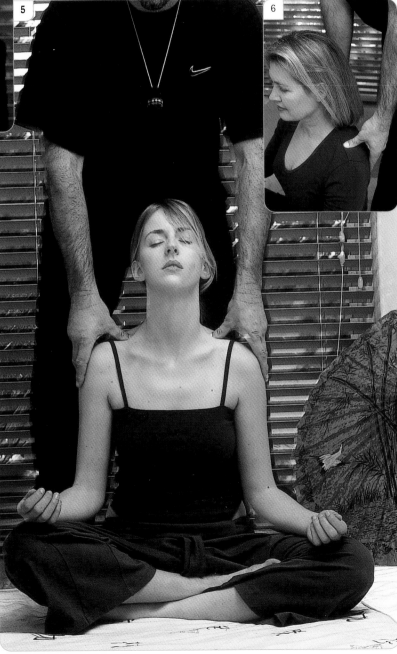

feedback. You may need to repeat this sequence a few times due to tension. The client can also turn her head from side to side on each thumb press. Finish off by repeating the palm presses to the same area, moving outward, then in.

This is a progression of the previous technique, except you're now using thumb presses, allowing you to concentrate more pressure into a smaller area — the trapezius muscles. You move outward through the three pressure points.

4 Begin with your thumbs positioned right next to the client's neck, your fingers pointing downward 5 toward her scapula. Ask the client to raise her head as you press down. You will find this allows far easier access into the muscle. To create the pressure through your thumbs, rock forward gently into each pressing movement. Hold pressure on each point for about five seconds.

6 Turn your hands to the front and work back to the neck on a parallel line to the one you have just worked on. This can be painful for the client, so ask for

ROCKING PALM PRESSES

Half-kneel behind your seated client. ☐1 Ask her to brace herself against the floor with straight arms. Palm press your way down her back alongside her spine. As both your hands are applying pressure at the same time, she will rock forward over her straight arms, while pushing her chest out and looking up.

Once you pass the centre of her back, fan your hands outward ☐2 and use butterfly palms.

Then, without your client rocking forward, do alternating palm presses up the back.

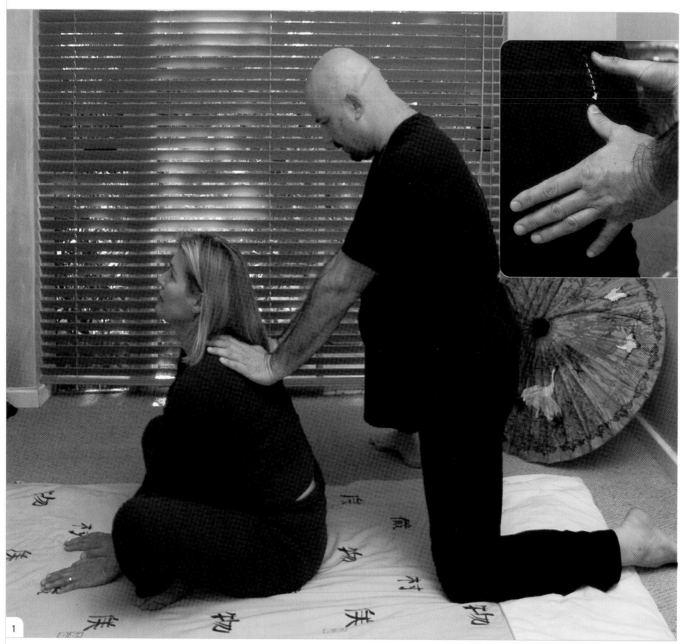

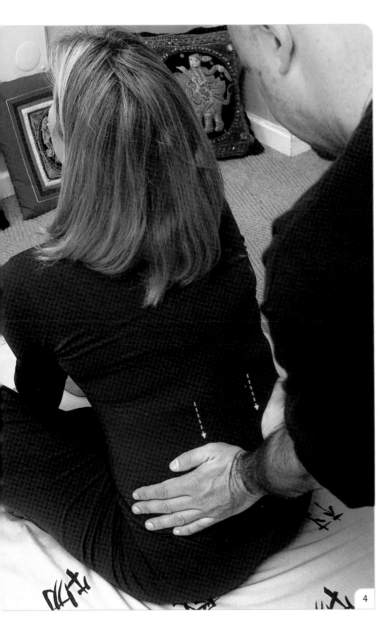

WAIST WORK

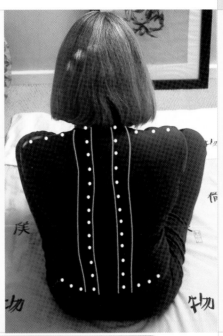

Indicated here are some of the energy lines, or meridians, running alongside the spine. Also illustrated are pressure points of the back, and points running across the top of the shoulders and horizontally at the waist.

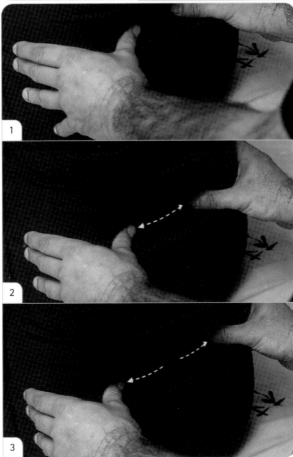

Repeat the previous technique, except this time use thumb presses. 1 – 3 When you reach the waist after thumb pressing down the back, apply thumb presses outward and inward in a 1-2-3-2-1 sequence to the four horizontal pressure points on the waist.

As before, the client rocks forward as you work down her back but not with the alternating thumb presses going up. 4 Finish off this technique by repeating the palm presses opposite.

SCAPULA RELEASE

[1] Fix one of your client's hands behind her back by pinning it there with your knee. [2] With one hand, pull her shoulder back, while the other hand warms up the scapula area with palm presses and palm circles. [3] Start working your way in under the edge of the scapula with thumb presses. Having done so, relax the area again with some palm circles. You can now use the hand that was supporting the shoulder to knead the arm down to the wrist and then up to the shoulder again. Carefully release her arm with a wide, semicircular movement.

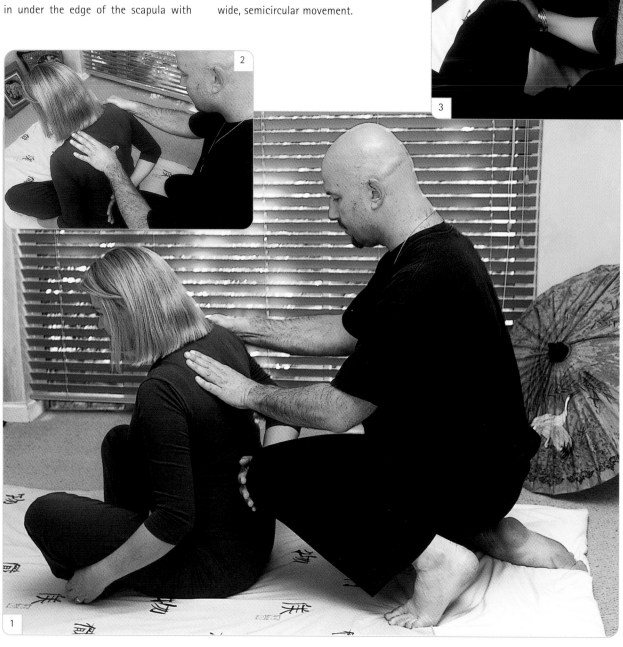

SHOULDER PRESSURE POINTS

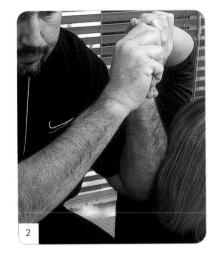

rests on her left shoulder and your left hand clasps her left wrist 3 while your right hand holds the fingers of her left hand.

There are three specific pressure points on each shoulder, as indicated in the photograph on p105. Position your elbow on the top point closest to the neck, work outward and down, then back the same

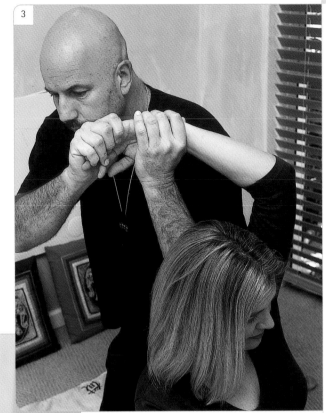

1 Half-kneel so that the other leg forms a 90-degree angle up against your client's back, supporting it. If your client is a woman, you work her left shoulder and arm first, with your left knee supporting her back. 2 Your left elbow

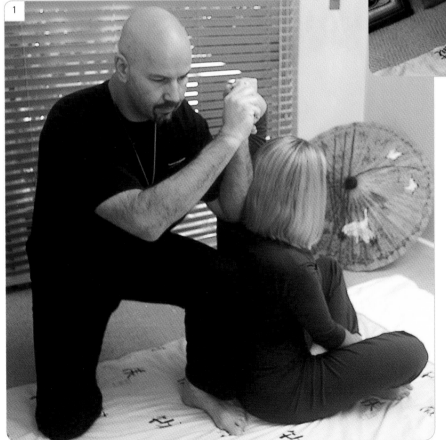

way again in a 1-2-3-2-1 sequence. As you place the tip of your elbow on the correct point, pull the client's arm and wrist with both hands while turning your trunk.

Apply this technique slowly, and constantly ask for feedback as you can apply a great deal of pressure into the points because of the leverage you have in this technique.

TRICEP RELEASE

Change your half-kneeling position, so that your other knee is now up alongside her body, with your body supporting her back. 1 Raise her right elbow and put her right hand on the back of her neck. Your left hand cups and supports her elbow, the other grasps her tricep, just above the armpit. 2 Pull back on the tricep muscle, turning your body to your right to create pressure. It is as if you are gently pulling the whole muscle off the bone. Move up and down the upper arm in a 1-2-3-2-1 sequence.

3 Next, you could knead the tricep itself with your fingers or with a loosely held fist you could use the 'chopping'

technique up and down the tricep. After opening the arm out, shake it gently.

Now repeat techniques 73 to 75 on the other arm.

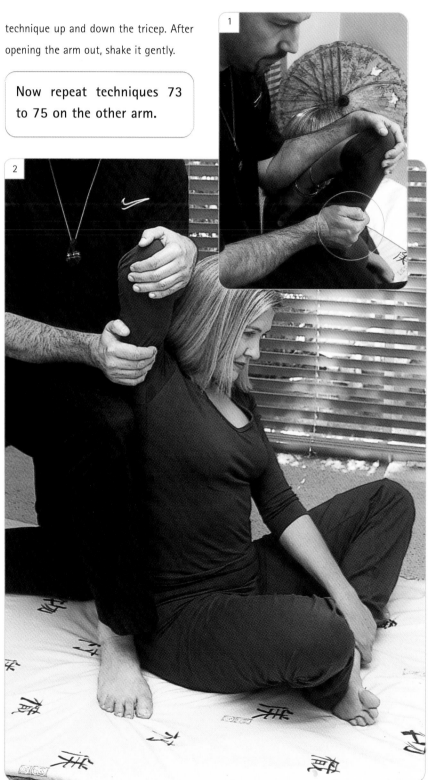

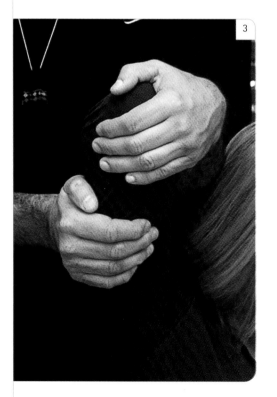

FOREARM NECK ROLL

Stand or kneel behind the client. Gently push her head to one side to open up the one shoulder and make it more accessible. 1 Hold her head in that position with either your hand or the forearm, just above her ear. 2 Now use your other forearm to 'iron out' the lower part of the neck and shoulder by rolling your forearm outward and pushing gently at the same time to stretch the muscle. Repeat this several times. Then apply the procedure to the other side.

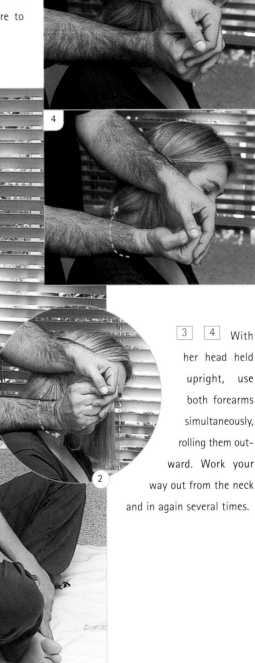

3 4 With her head held upright, use both forearms simultaneously, rolling them outward. Work your way out from the neck and in again several times.

NECK PALM PRESSES

First warm up the neck. Place your hands on your client's shoulders and do thumb circles with the thumbs, pressing into and kneading the muscle. You can also use finger circles for this purpose. As an option, support the client's forehead with one hand, using the fingers and thumb of the other hand as a clamp to warm up the neck.

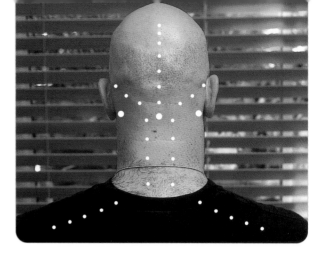

Above: **The main pressure points of the back of the scalp, neck and shoulders.**

Now ask the client to tilt her head forward. ☐1 Interlace your fingers and squeeze her neck with your palms, starting at the base of the neck and working your way up to the ☐2 occiput (base of the skull), then working back down again. Repeat this a few times.

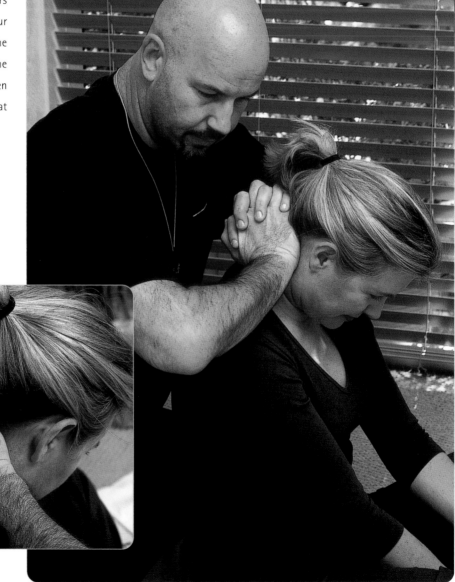

NECK THUMB PRESSES

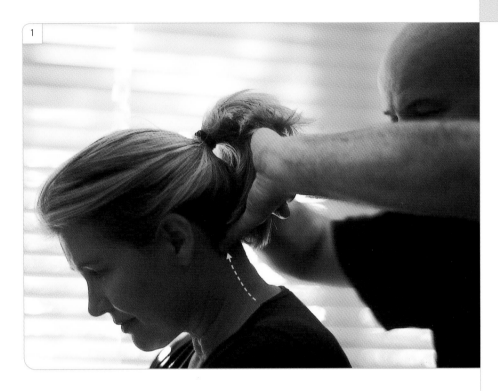

This is essentially the same technique you have just done with your palms, but this time you apply thumb presses. ⬜1 With fingers interlaced and hands angled toward the back of the head to better access the neck, extend your thumbs and press them to either side of her upper neck. ⬜2 ⬜3 Work your way up and then down the neck a few times. The pressure for this technique comes from the butterfly action of the elbows. Do this gently, as you are concentrating a lot of force into a small area.

To finish off, do the palm squeeze of the previous technique up and down the neck a few times, then do some generalized pressing and kneading. End up just below the client's occiput, as this is where the next technique starts.

These two techniques are also very useful for you personally, as the practitioner. If you do several massages every day, you'll end up with your own aches and pains. Interlace your fingers, put your arms behind your head with your palms on your neck, tilt your head forward a little and work your way up and down the neck. When you feel it has been warmed up sufficiently, use your thumbs in the same way as described opposite for your client.

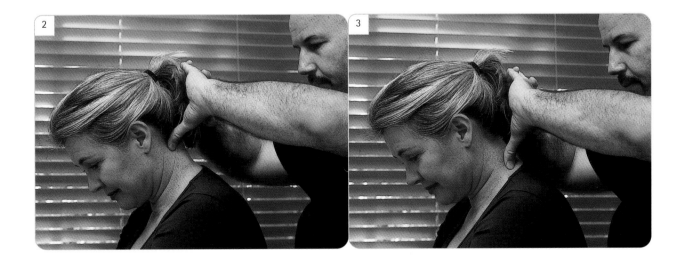

DOUBLE FOREARM ROLL

While half-kneeling behind your client, who is seated upright, relax her shoulders by kneading and applying finger circles over the trapezius muscle. 1 Placing your forearms to either side of her neck, roll them outward over the shoulder, using the portion of forearm that's closer to the elbow. 2 Three or four such rolling movements should get you to the bony outer part of the shoulder; work your way back to the neck with the same motion.

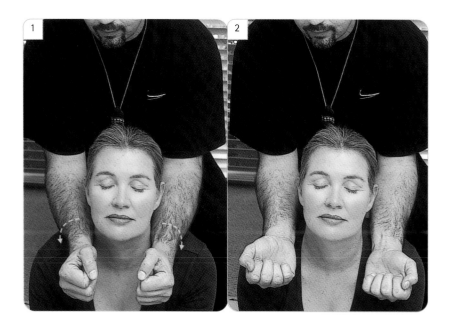

Now place your hands in the prayer position so that your client can rest her chin on the base of your thumbs. 3 She braces herself on the floor with fully extended arms as you rock forward in your kneeling stance and she in turn rocks over her arms, pushing her chest forward. The placement of your arms lifts her head up and works as a stretch for the neck. 4 Rock back and repeat, this time guiding her head so that she is looking to one side. 5 Rock back and repeat to the other side. Do one last forward rock, lifting the head straight up once more (1-2-3-1). Finish with some finger circles on the shoulders.

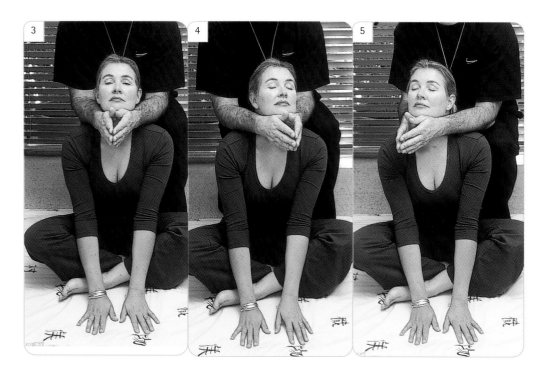

Note that you are not lifting her head by exerting pressure with your arm muscles. They serve merely as a convenient lever; it is the rocking motion that fluidly and gently moves the head and facilitates the stretch.

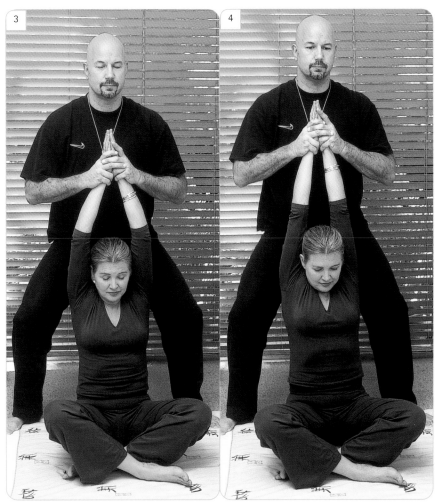

RIBCAGE STRETCH

1 Stand behind the client, supporting her back with the outside of your leg. Ask the client to interlace her fingers and put her hands behind her head. Cup each of her elbows with one of your hands.

2 Pull back on her elbows and slightly lift. This gives the movement a bit of an upward curve. Do the stretch three times, first gently, fairly strongly the second time, and gently to finish.

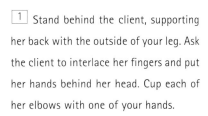

Since you are slightly side-on to the client, your pulling action may be a bit uneven, favouring one side. To correct this, simply switch legs and repeat on the other side.

3 Now ask the client to extend both arms straight above her head, hands together in the prayer position. Bend your legs. 4 Hold her wrists and, straightening your legs, lift her briefly off the floor. Remember to use your leg muscles to lift her; never bend your back as you do this, you will injure yourself. If your client is larger or heavier than yourself, you may want to leave out this technique.

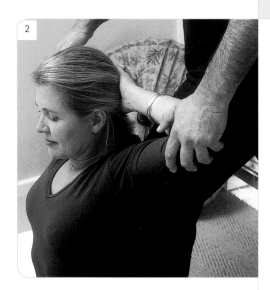

SPINAL RELEASE

Half-kneel behind the client. Place your one knee next to her floating ribs, while the front of your thigh of the other leg supports her back. She interlaces her fingers and rests her hands behind her head. 1 Threading your arms under her armpits, 2 place your hands against her forearms. Push her head forward toward her feet, then pull her up again.

Use the thigh that is supporting her back to press forward as you pull her up vertically. This creates a nice counter-stretch for her spine.

Repeat the procedure three times. Relax your fingers between each repetition, otherwise you could cause neck pain for the client.

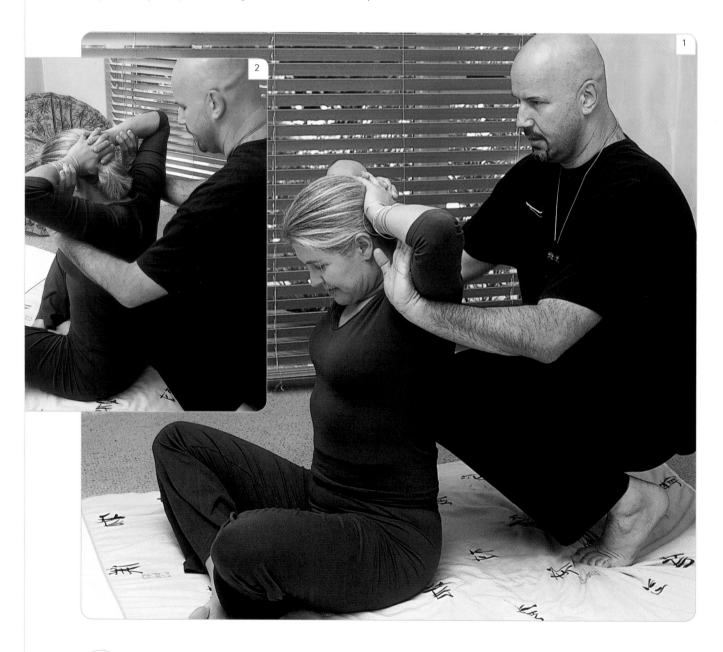

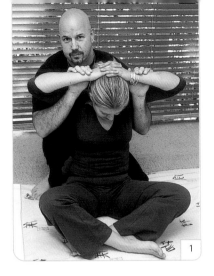

SPINAL ROTATION

This is a rotational stretch for the spine. Your client is in the same position as opposite, except that you use your knee on her upper thigh, or a straight leg draped over it, to hold her in position.

[1] Thread your arms through as in the previous technique and [2] twist your client away from the side that's secured by your knee. If you hear a 'popping' sound in her spine, stop. It does not signify that anything's wrong; it's simply an indication that you've achieved what you set out to do with the technique.

If this does not occur, move your knee forward, closer to the middle of her thigh and repeat the stretch. Then move your knee even closer to her knee and repeat once more. As you move your knee forward on her thigh, you're no longer fixing her position with your thigh and bracing her back, so it allows a greater range of motion. After the third twist, return her torso to the centre, then do one repetition of the technique opposite,

[3] a forward and upward stretch. Repeat the three stretches on the other side, and finish with a forward stretch.

It is very important that you do this technique slowly and fluidly. Never exert force suddenly or in a jerky manner when doing any work involving the spine.

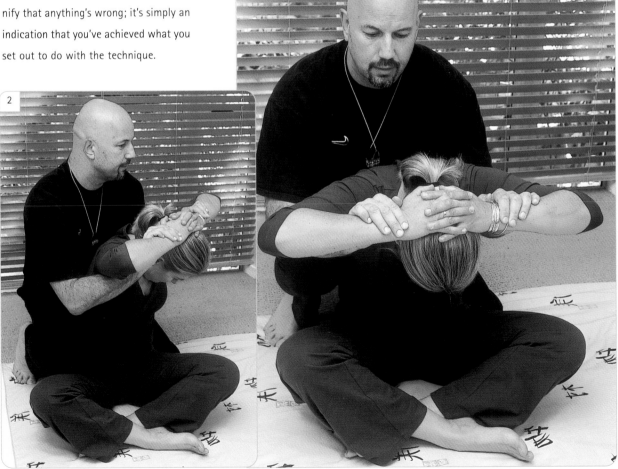

PROCEDURE 84

SPINAL WALK

Sit behind the client. 1 Ask her to extend her arms straight out behind her. Take hold of her forearms; she can also grasp your wrist. 2 Place your feet against her lower back, and gently walk up and down the back, to either side of her spine. Your client assists the technique by gently raising her chest.

3 You create the pressure by bending and extending your legs, not by pulling on her arms.

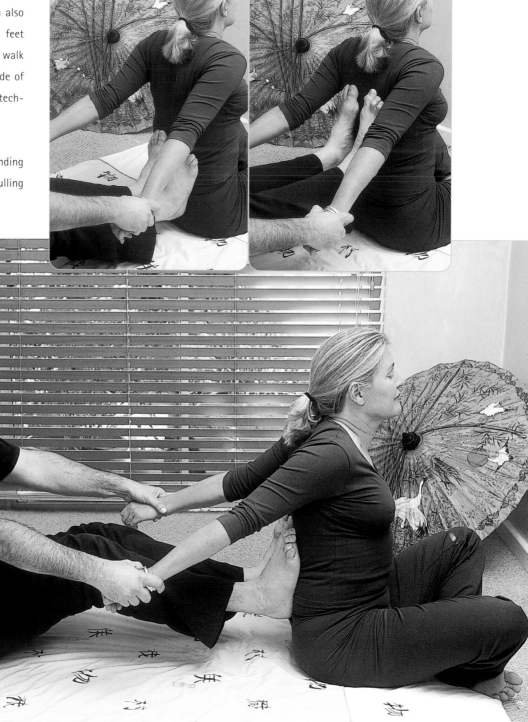

SPINAL STRETCH

1 Ask your client to cross her arms and wrap them around her chest, placing one palm just under her armpit on the opposite side of her body, the other palm on the outside of her opposite shoulder.

2 Squat behind her, placing your knees against her lower back, to either side of the spine, and take hold of her hands. Now create pressure by leaning back with your upper body. Then move your knees a few inches up from the first spot and repeat. Return to the original spot and do it one last time.

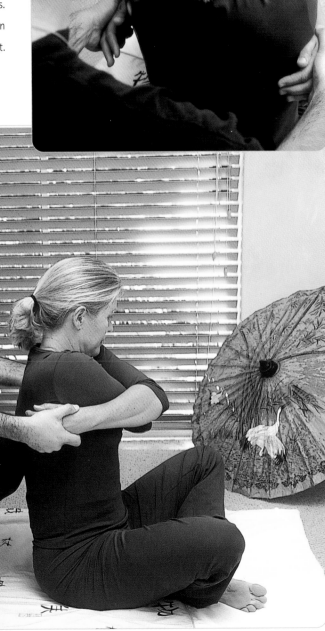

LOWER BACK ROTATION

Stand next to your seated client. If you're tall, you may be able to apply this technique in the half-kneeling position. Your client cups one ear with her hand while you cup the elbow of the same arm. Grasp her forearm with your other hand; she can take hold of your wrist. 1 Hold her knee in position with your foot.

2 By pushing against her elbow and simultaneously pulling on her opposite arm, you effect a rotational stretch for the lower back.

Repeat this procedure on the other side.

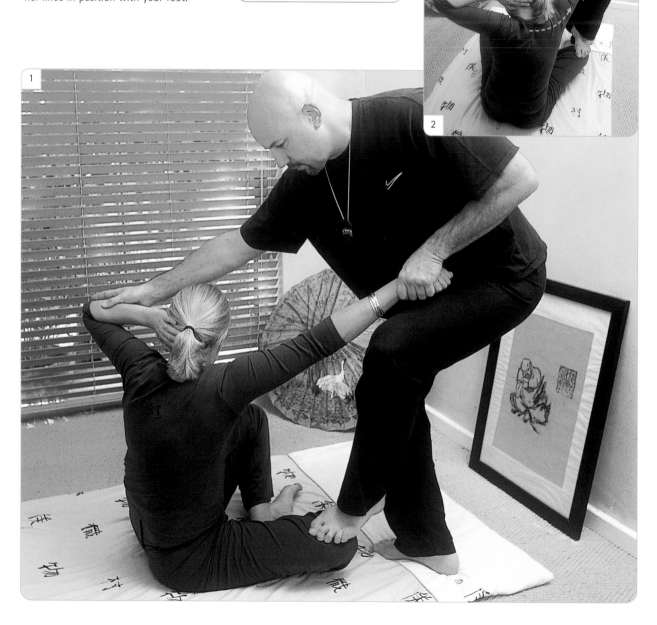

BUTTERFLY PRESSES TO BACK

The client is seated upright and braces herself against the mat with straight arms (not illustrated here, see procedure 104, p71). Palm press down the back to either side of the spine, using both hands together. When you get to the mid-back, turn your hands out and use butterfly palms. Finish with alternating palm presses going up the back.

If your client is supple, you could gently press her torso forward to the floor from her cross-legged seated position. Otherwise, ask the client to ☐1 kneel and lean forward, putting her forehead and forearms on the mat. Do the 'X' stretch diagonally across her back as in procedure 68, p99.

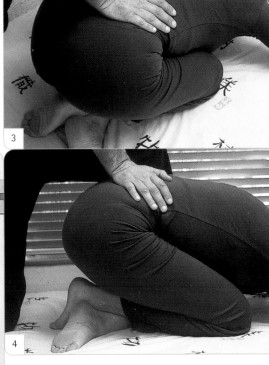

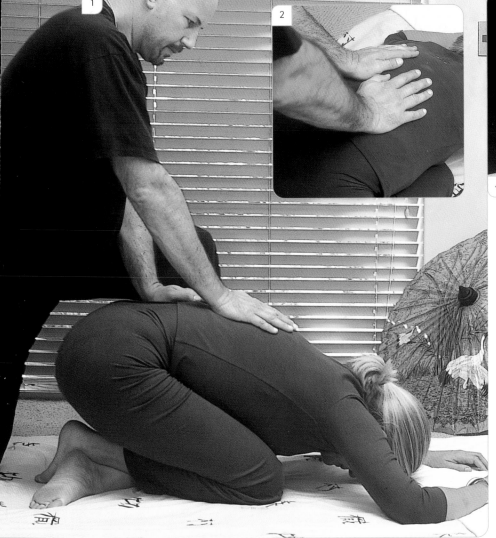

While the client is in this position, do palm presses down the back with hands together, then up with ☐2 alternating hands, changing to ☐3 ☐4 butterfly palms at the mid-back.

Have the client sit up cross-legged again. Knead her shoulders, then finish with the double-handed chopping technique on the sides of the neck, the shoulders and the back. To close off the work for the seated position, lightly brush down your client's arms and back with your hands.

SCALP THUMB PRESSES

1 Once more get into a half-kneeling position, the shin of your one leg supporting your client's back. Support the head by holding her forehead with one hand. If you work the energy lines and pressure points on the back of the head without simultaneously countering the pressure from the front, the strain on her neck will be counterproductive. Work the horizontal line of the pressure points below the occiput.

2 You can be creative working the scalp and facial area, making use of thumb circles, finger circles or even the tips of several fingers simultaneously — with your fingers both together and apart.

3a 3b Work the centreline of the skull, starting at the last vertebra of the spine and running to the forehead, using thumb presses. You can either try 4 walking alternate thumb presses or you can put one thumb on top of the other, using them together to create added pressure.

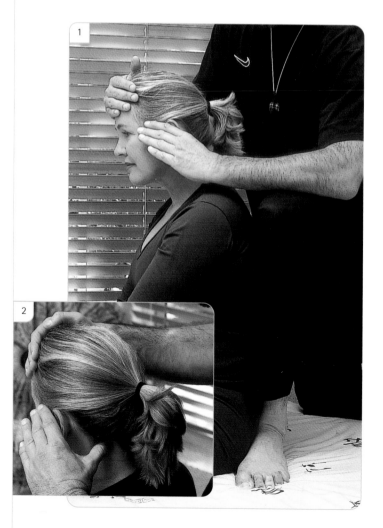

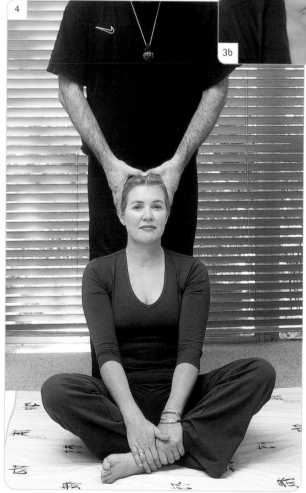

CLOSING OFF THE MASSAGE

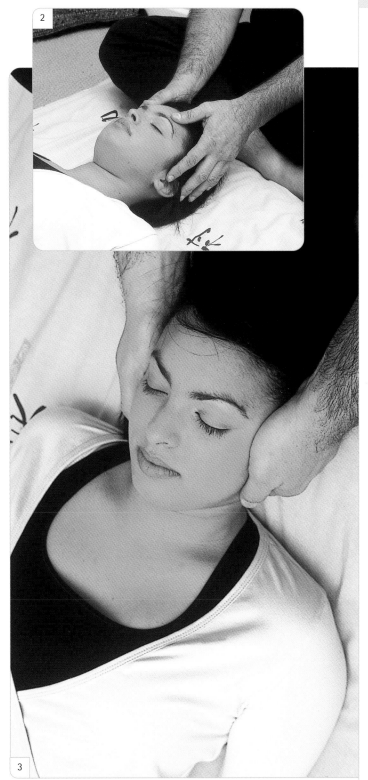

To close off the massage, ask your client to once again lie on her back. This is the part of the massage that people generally enjoy the most. You can spend some time working into the shoulders (trapezius) using your thumbs. Then, with your fingers, work the neck muscles to either side of the spine.

Gently massage the entire scalp area, as if you were working shampoo into the client's hair. Apply thumb presses to the centreline from the forehead to the back of the scalp.

Once you have finished massaging the scalp, make a smooth transition into a facial massage. 1 2 Start with the thumbs touching in the middle of the forehead and brush outward. Do finger circles on the temples, the hinges of the jaw and the chin area. Lightly pull and massage the ears.

3 To finish the massage, cover both of the client's ears with your cupped hands for anything up to a minute. This has a deeply relaxing effect on most people. Some may even fall asleep while you are doing this.

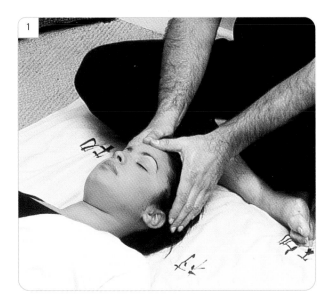

CLIENT QUESTIONNAIRE

Full name

Date of birth

Height

Weight

Sex

Address

Telephone   (H)

                   (W)

Mobile phone

E-mail

Date of treatment

Your state of health

Reasons for seeking treatment

You were referred by/heard about Thai massage from?

Your current medications (if any)

Any chronic medical conditions/health problems?

Are you menstruating?

Are you pregnant? If so, how many weeks?

Please list any recent major operations/surgery

Are you particularly stiff in any of your joints i.e. are there any yoga stretches/postures that may cause you pain/discomfort?

_____

Do you suffer from (or have you experienced in the past) any neck or back pain?

_____

What type of exercise, if any, do you engage in?

_____

_____

What do you hope Thai massage will do for you?

_____

_____

_____

Important: Do you suffer from one or more of the following conditions?

◯ Allergies	◯ Haemophilia	◯ Osteoporosis
◯ Skin disease	◯ Open wounds and cuts	◯ Joint problems
◯ Migraine/headaches	◯ Phlebitis	◯ Rheumatoid arthritis
◯ Fever	◯ Arteriosclerosis	◯ Old/new bone fractures
◯ Diabetes	◯ Stroke	◯ Previous dislocation
◯ Diarrhoea	◯ Varicose veins	◯ Cancer
◯ Constipation	◯ Heart disease	◯ AIDS
◯ Hernia	◯ Strained, sprained or torn muscles	◯ Any other not listed here
◯ High blood pressure	◯ Cervical spine problems	

CLIENT QUESTIONNAIRE – PATIENT'S CONSENT

Patient consent

I understand that the intent of Thai massage is to aid the prevention of health problems and induce a general state of relaxation. It is not to be considered a diagnosis of any illness, disease or physical disorder or condition. I have honestly represented my personal state of health here and not withheld any pertinent information from my Thai massage practitioner.

Client signature   date

Thai massage practitioner's observations

Contraindications (if any)

Areas needing special care

Sensitive/stiff areas

Additional notes

Length of session

Further reading and contacts

Apfelbaum, Ananda (2004) *Thai Massage: Sacred Bodywork.* Avery: New York.

Baloti Lawrence, D; Harrison, Lewis (1983) *Massage Works.* Penguin/Putnam Publishing Co.: New York.

Brust, Harald (Asokananda) (1993) *The Art of Traditional Thai Massage.* Editions Duang Kamol.

Claire, Thomas (1995) *Body Work.* Quill/William Morrow: New York.

Gerber, Richard (1988) *Vibrational Medicine.* Bear & Company: Santa Fe, New Mexico.

Gold, Richard (2003) *Thai Massage: A Traditional Medical Technique.* Churchill Livingstone: Philadelphia.

Kam Thye Chow (2004) *Thai Yoga Massage.* Healing Arts Press: Rochester, Vermont.

Kira Balaskas (2002) *Thai Yoga Massage.* Thorsons: London.

Lambert, Arthur with Setthakorn, Chongkol (1993) *Nuad Bo-Rarn, The Ancient Massage of Thailand.* Institute of Thai Massage: Chiang Mai, Thailand.

Rynerson, Kay (2001) *Thai Massage Workbook.* Kay Rynerson: Seattle.

Sombat Tapanya (1993) *Traditional Thai Massage.* Editions Duang Kamol, Bangkok.

Contacts

Institute of Thai Massage (Chongkol Setthakorn), 17/7 Morakot Road, Hah Yaek Santhitham, Chiang Mai, Thailand 50300.
Tel: +66-53-218632;
website: thaimassage.org

Wat Po Thai Traditional Massage School, Sanamchai Road, Wat Po, Bangkok 10200.
Tel: +66-2-2254771 / 2212874

Foundation of Shivago Komarpaj,
Old Medicine Hospital, 78/1 Wualai Road, Chiang Mai, Thailand.
Tel: +66-53-275085
149, Kaew Nawarat Soi 4 (Asokananda/Harald Brust), Chiang Mai 50300, Thailand.
e-mail: asokasunshine@hotmail.com;
website: thaiyogamassage.infothai.com

International Professional School of Body Work (Richard Gold), Pacific College of Oriental Medicine, San Diego, CA, USA.
e-mail: rmgold@znet.com

Traditional Thai Massage Center (Ananda Apfelbaum), 92 Foster Street, Littleton, MA 01460, USA.
Tel: +1-978-4863440;
e-mail: ananda@traditionalthaiyoga-massage.com;
website: www.traditionalthaiyogamassage.com

The School of Thai Yoga Massage (Kira Balaskas), PO Box 33822, London N8 8XA.
e-mail: info@thaiyogamassage.co.uk;
website: www.thaiyogamassage.co.ukself-massage

The London School of Thai Massage (Simon Gall).
Tel: +44-020-84601213;
e-mail: info@lstm.co.uk;
website: www.lstm.co.uk

INDEX